Longing for Nothingness

Longing for Nothingness

Resistance, Denial, and the Place of Death in the Nursing Home

Andrew Stein

JASON ARONSON
Lanham • Boulder • New York • Toronto • Plymouth, UK

Published by Jason Aronson
An imprint of Rowman & Littlefield Publishers, Inc.
A wholly owned subsidiary of The Rowman & Littlefield Publishing Group, Inc.
4501 Forbes Boulevard, Suite 200, Lanham, Maryland 20706
http://www.rowmanlittlefield.com

Estover Road, Plymouth PL6 7PY, United Kingdom

British Library Cataloguing in Publication Information Available

Library of Congress Cataloging-in-Publication Data

Stein, Andrew, 1959–
Longing for nothingness : resistance, denial, and the place of death in the nursing home / Andrew Stein.
p. cm.
Includes bibliographical references and index.
ISBN 978-0-7657-0577-8 (cloth : alk. paper)
ISBN 978-0-7657-0578-5 (electronic)
1. Death—Psychological aspects. 2. Nursing home patients—Psychology. 3. Nursing homes—Psychological aspects. 4. Chronic diseases—Psychological aspects. I. Title.
BF789.D4S72 2010
155.9'37—dc22 2009038487

∞™ The paper used in this publication meets the minimum requirements of American National Standard for Information Sciences—Permanence of Paper for Printed Library Materials, ANSI/NISO Z39.48-1992.

Printed in the United States of America

Contents

Acknowledgments

This book never would have been written without the support and guidance of a number of people. Chief among these is Aaron Bender, who has been a kind of spiritual guide through most of the period that I conceived, planned, and wrote this book. Also, I want to acknowledge the support given me by Leslie Rosenthal, Curtis Bowman, Thomas Prasch, and the entire *Aprés Coup* group in New York City, who graciously put up with my commentaries and questions for a very long time. Finally, I wish to thank the residents and staff at the various nursing homes and adult centers with whom I work. They are the real teachers. All opinions presented in this book are my own.

Part I

DEATH AND THE CHAIN OF LIFE

1

The Destructive Side of Our Erotic Life

> A little poison now and then: that makes for pleasant dreams. And much poison at the end, for a pleasant death. They have their little pleasures for the day, and their little pleasures for the night, but they have a regard for health. "We have discovered happiness," says the Last Men, and they blink.
>
> —Frederick Nietzsche, *Thus Spoke Zarathustra*

It took me a long time to figure out what this book would be about. I knew I wanted to write about my experience working with residents in nursing homes, many of whom are anxious about dying or are death obsessed. Death plays a huge role in their fantasies—a vast field of fears, longings, resignations, paranoias, and aggressions masking elemental questions about their mortality and the mortality of the people they love and hate. They have all lost loved ones whose absence is inconsolable; most are depressed by health problems. Many are absorbed with knowing when enough is enough and, depending on their character and circumstance, wish to live or die. Often these struggles with mortality do not rise to the level of consciousness at all but go on in the preconscious and unconscious zones and have to be unmasked in the presentations of dreams and symptoms. Death and thoughts of death are, in any case, never far below the surface. Death becomes the great point around which their inner lives turn. They seem to constantly be circling it like a dream circles around an enigma. I had my topic: death obsessions.

While wondering how to organize this material, I knew I did not want to write a phenomenology of death. However interesting, a study of the consciousness of death would only describe the outer works of a vaster subject—the unconscious obsession with death.[1] I decided to look at what others had written about the topic. The themes of preconscious and unconscious love and death obsession have always found a home in literature. Hamlet and many of Shakespeare's other memorable characters are death obsessed, of course. But from Yorick's skull to Kafka's bug, death obsession appears in modern tragic and comic literature as an endless fountain for fate or farce. Poetry too has been welcoming to the theme. At a poetry reading, Alan Ginsberg spoke of the importance of death for poets and then demonstrated the point by reciting the opening pages of his "Kaddish" poem about his deceased mother and his remembrance of the lost world of her childhood, of her coming to America, of the family, and of her madness and death. But religion and philosophy have been the most death obsessed in both the ancient and modern worlds. The late ancient world was saturated by philosophic mystery cults like the Elysian mysteries of Demeter and her daughter Persephone, who was taken by the god of the underworld and which is an allegory of death and rebirth specifically of the return to the One by the purified soul after death, like the Stoic and Epicurean philosophers who learned to embrace the inevitable, to control their passions, and to accept death; and Christianity, of course, is a religion which promises to conquer death. In the modern era, too, political theory has turned on the problem of the artful control of human violence while Darwinism has had its say about the dialectic of adaptation and death in the evolution of the species.

In other words, every area of knowledge and desire has addressed the obsession with death and violence. Art, philosophy, religion, political theory, and science, all the varieties of human imagination and knowledge have proven in turn to be death obsessed. But it was by searching into Freud's dual-drive theory, a much maligned and in some quarters all but forgotten meta-theory about how life and the neuroses form out of the clash of life and death drives, that I discovered my way into this material.

Let me in a very cursory way situate Freud's second dual-drive theory in the history of psychoanalysis. This second or dual-drive theory became Freud's central meta-theory for the last twenty years of his life, but the majority of analysts did not follow Freud down this path. Many analysts opposed the idea from the start. Moreover, the dissenters, who quickly outnumbered the supporters, included Wilhelm Reich and Heinz Hartman—a more eclectic group of analysts you could not imagine. The supporters too, who included Ferenczi, Klein, Lacan, and Eisler, and who were also an eclectic lot, quickly converted the death drive to fit into their own systems, which increasingly looked less and less as Freud had imagined things should look.

Most of the ego psychologists who dominated the APA after World War II either opposed the idea or relegated it to a side (if honored) bar. With a few noteworthy exceptions, the suggestion that people have death obsessed unconscious erotic lives did not sit well with the postwar spirit of consumerism and superficial optimism when the problem before people was how to push the horrors of the war, the recent "discovery" of the holocaust, the terror of a nuclear winter, and a post-apocalyptic future to one side and cash in on the postwar consumer optimism boom. In this climate, no one wanted to seriously consider that normal folks are death obsessed or capable of acts of utter depravity and destruction as the dual-drive theory implies—in the mood of escapism and optimism such anxieties were transformed into entertainment like *Psycho*, *The Three Faces of Eve*, and *The Manchurian Candidate*, or relegated to the analyst's couch. Ego psychologists performed an historic and cultural role by supporting socially normative values that did not scare or disturb most people while promoting a certain fascination with the derangements that could befall "abnormal" minds.

Ego psychology, therefore, leads to a very different view of human nature and the possibility of human depravity than dual-drive theory. Besides rejecting the notion that normal people are motivated to destroy as much as love, Hartman, Lowenstein, et al. wanted to strengthen what Hartman called the nonconflictual zones of mental life. Moreover, Hartman et al. wanted to make psychoanalysis the center of a more general psychology with normative values concerning what constitutes mental health and sickness by integrating psychoanalysis with academic psychology and the social sciences.

By the sixties and seventies the dominance of ego psychology was on the wane.[2] Challenged by new therapies developing within psychoanalysis (self psychology was one example, the explosion of interest in Lacanian psychoanalysis was another) and without (the new humanist, existential, logotherapies, and so on), the hegemony of the Hartman era was also disputed by analysts who called for a more clinic-centered psychoanalytic literature and developed an aversion to the theory building of Hartman et al. This aversion arose out of a growing criticism that clinical and metapsychological knowledge did not correlate with each other anymore. I suspect that what was going on was that some analysts were waking up to the fact that Freud's and Hartman's meta-theories had their roots in a European culture that existed before World War II (although Hartman adapted it to postwar American culture) and which increasingly was felt to be out of touch with the new American century and Cold War conflicts that had just begun. It goes without saying that in such a climate dual-drive theory was discussed less and less, for to dwell on the human potential for destruction reminded many of European existential despair—people had had quite enough of that.[3]

Although it actually came late, this turn from theory to empirically driven, clinically near knowledge piggy-backed on wider cultural changes in some areas of the social and human sciences after World War II in America. Thus, while some social scientific writing became overtly more political—especially sociological studies of postwar prosperity—twentieth-century scientific empiricism gained ascendancy in other areas of the social sciences.[4] This claimed to be apolitical and neutral but in fact was anything but, and therefore, although they were unaware of the fact, the turn toward clinically near knowledge was a piece of a general Cold War assault on ideological (read Marxist) knowledge;[5] and, again, although the proponents of clinic-centered knowledge and practice did not know this, their empiricism presumed a synthesis between two ideals in line with the ideology of a triumphant Western-branded capitalism: the ideal of postwar prosperity as a road to personal happiness and a democratic society and the ideal of scientific neutrality as road to a Truth beyond ideology or the self-interest of the truth-seeker.

The problem was that knowledge cannot be neutral, especially in a century as ideological as the twentieth century, and, speaking epistemologically, swearing off metapsychology does not do away with the need for basic organizing principles to make sense of clinically driven knowledge anymore than an emphasis on emotionally corrective experiences à la Ferenczi, Balint, and Winnicott (especially important when working with regressed patients) frees the analyst from the obligation of making corrective interpretation before an analysis is complete. Thus, when Gill and others wrote about transference dynamics in the clinic they willy-nilly brought in metapsychological explanations whether these explanations were analyzed or left hanging.

At the other extreme, a new political and cultural radicalism made its effect felt in the psychoanalytic movement at about the same time. While some radical ideas came from analysts who were hold outs from the Old Left (see the *rundebriefen* between Fenichel, Reich, Jacobson, Eichhorn, and so on),[6] that radical tradition had been squashed in Europe and America. A new political and cultural radicalism arose around the ideals of the New Left, however, based in Reichian slogans of a return to nature and sexual liberation. The New Left critique of social alienation also fueled the Frankfurt School liberation philosophy of Marcuse. In books like *Eros and Civilization*, Marcuse linked Freud's theory of repression and Marx's discussion of surplus value added to the labor of the proletariat to generate a new concept of a revolutionary surplus pleasure.[7] Needless to say, both Reichian and Marcusian liberation ideologies were optimistic philosophies that could make little sense out of Freud's discussion of the death-obsessed unconscious erotic lives of people.[8] Reich in particular had led the challenge to the death drive theory in his day because it contradicted his view that the neuroses are the psychological sicknesses of Capitalist and Fascist societies enforcing an authoritarian personality and his vision of the revolutionary potential of liberated sexuality (Eros).

In the long run, however, the women's and gay liberation movements have had a greater influence on American psychoanalysis than either the New Left or the empiricism of the sixties and seventies. But both the women's and the gay rights movements were originally suspicious of psychoanalysis, which they regarded as a pillar of the establishment and the male-centered status quo that stood in the way of women entering the work place and gays winning equal rights with heterosexuals; and, as a result, the analysts influenced by these great social and cultural movements of the second half of the twentieth century made Freud a target of severe criticism or outright forgetting. That ego psychology was the real target of their criticisms was lost on almost all of Freud's critics at first. So, too, was the fact that many younger gay and women activists in America and Europe (to varying degrees) began turning to psychoanalysis in less critical ways. Thus, even though writers continued to treat Freud as a dead European white guy who had to be cleared out of the way, many of his ideas in combination with new ideas from the gay and women's rights movements crept back into their writings. A feminist reading of Lacan was an early example of this shift.[9] Irigary's celebration of semiotic discourse beyond the restrictions of castrated signifiers and patriarchically driven chains of signifiers also point to an alliance between Freudians and feminists and is a serious effort to develop a feminist psychoanalytic theory of language and literature.[10]

Both Irigaray and Lacan, at least the Lacan after 1972, that is the "later Lacan" who alters his (Freudian) belief that there is only one kind of libido so he can entertain the possibility of another, evanescent, contingent, always fleeting "feminine sexuality," and an "other *jouissance,*" that (much like the object a) is both in and transgresses the order of "phallic *jouissance*" of the Symbolic that Lacan associates with "masculine sexuality." And, yet, although these are discourses on the "possible, impossible, contingent, and universal" modes of representing libido and sexuality, both Irigaray and Lacan treat death as an event-horizon where the Symbolic breaks down as it approaches "the impossible." In other words, this mode of the "impossible," which signifies a forbidden "beyond" of phallic *jouissance* and the Symbolic order, is, at least for Lacan, a world patrolled by death, especially the death drive. Thus, at the event-horizon of the Symbolic, that is at the event-horizon of the human world, the world transformed by speech and language (man is the *parlétre*—the speaking being, for Lacan, who, therefore, is cut off from the "natural" sexuality and *jouissance* of the rest of the animal world), knowledge always fails to measure up to a truth (there is something forbidden and left out that is somehow connected to a forbidden *jouissance*) where death and the forbidden marks the passage to a utopian post-Symbolic where the "sign of the father" or patriarchal categories no longer reign.[11]

For others, an encounter with death at the limit of the Symbolic has quasi-religious overtones connoting the "surreal marvelous" covered over like a tomb by the Symbolic.[12] But we can be sure of one thing: even if we are able to reach a post-patriarchal semiotic, death would follow us there and would still produce neuroses in need of treatment.

And that is why the approach to a forbidden zone beyond language is always bound to death. In her own, quite different way, Melanie Klein will also explore this world of death drives that exist before language and at the moment before language and the ego are securely rooted in the psyche of the child; and she will find there (I mean especially in the later) a world of unconscious fantasy and of self and other-destructive defenses that are only slowly (and never completely) modified by the child's development of a richer object relations world. Lacan and Klein will both be discussed in subsequent chapters where Lacan's *object* a (of the gaze, and so on)—the lost object of the Real—will be examined as a bridge between the Real, the Imaginary, the Symbolic, and death.

The postmodern influence on American psychoanalysis since the 1980s has been nearly as great as the women's and gay liberation movement's influence on it. But what is postmodernism? The word is bantered about so much we scarcely recognize how poorly it is defined. Postmodernism has been called the cultural equivalent to democratic globalization, but its original association with an architecture that combined styles from different regions and periods of the world has all but been forgotten due to postmodernism's complex history as an intellectual movement.

Postmodernism emerged in the sixties in part as a reaction to a number of intellectual trends, in particular the epistemological dominance of so-called objective knowledge in the sciences, the existential phenomenology of Hegel (à la Kojeve), Heidegger, and Sartre, a new global cultural politics that embraced difference as its guiding star, and the slow-dawning on the Left of the failings of totalitarian Communism. A highly complicated, culturally heterodox, and often contradictory movement, postmodernism celebrates multiplicity and difference and critiques binary, dialectic, and universalizing forms of knowledge. In its textual analysis, postmodernism opens the text (which everything now is presumed to be) to multiple, heterodox meanings and readings, and like its cousin deconstruction, it explodes the idea that a text has a central author and meaning (that an expert can explicate).

Postmodern writers treat literature less as a privileged window into immutable if unconscious or hidden truths than as a revolutionary battering ram to knock down the concept and the subject, and to replace them with the overflow of excess.[13] Thus, rather than signify a reality seen darkly through our senses and reason, the idea becomes that: "Language engenders the thing."[14]

All roads, then, do not lead to Rome because Rome is only a signifier. Hence, postmodernism like its sister post-structuralism is deeply antithetical to the Socratic and Platonic theory of knowledge; and it tends to see those seeking the Truth as deluding themselves or having a secret—or not so secret—totalitarian agenda. In politics, postmodernism celebrates multiplicity and the disintegration of centralized power symbolically linked to the tyranny of reason, and it embraces a noncentralized political culture that is deeply sympathetic to democratic liberation movements around the world, subaltern revolts, and third wave feminist's sensitivity to women of different classes, races, ages, and so on, as well as to the varieties of gender and sexual roles that women and men can occupy.[15]

As a result, analysts influenced by postmodernism celebrate diversity and difference, and they have played a role in problematizing the diagnoses of homosexuality and transgender differences.[16] When they take any interest in Freud at all, postmodernists celebrate him for decentering the subject and showing that humans are not the masters of their own minds. More frequently, they vilify him for imposing his own *idées fixes* on his followers or for distorting sexuality and gender categories. Postmodernism, however, suffers from over-stylized views of death, too. To the degree that postmodernism is another liberation ideology, it does not analyze Freud's gloomier side of how death, violence, and destructive fantasies dominate life.

A new group of psychoanalytic schools have emerged in America in the last thirty years. Collectively, they go by the name of relational, interpersonal, or intersubjective psychology. Because of their number and variety, it is ultimately of limited value to make sweeping claims about them except to say that the relational schools criticize Freud for believing in objective knowledge which supposedly proves he did not appreciate that people are psychologically sustained in social or relational matrices and that the role of the analyst is to help patients navigate these (partly co-created) matrices in the same (or an analogous) way that a mother does with her newborn infant; as a result, relational psychologists emphasize emotionally corrective experiences à la Ferenczi, Balint, and Winnicott over interpretation. Currently "on the rise," they also reflect a cultural *zeitgeist* of late Capitalism just as ego psychology mirrored a *zeitgeist* of the post–World War II Cold War era.[17] The current *zeitgeist*, however, downplays the individual (Christopher Lasch's

The Culture of Narcissism[18] already prophesied these trends in the seventies) even as it stresses her existence in relational matrices or networks. Thus, just as in the sixties it was Freud's fate to be lambasted as a pillar of patriarchy when he had done as much as anyone in his time to question the psychological foundation of patriarchy, so, too, it has been his fate to be lambasted by the relational schools for developing a one-person psychology when he did as much as anyone in his day to question the psychological foundations of the individual (even though he wanted people to become more mature individuals living with others in a common universal culture).

A response to the relational schools would point out Aron et al.'s over-simplified views about the incompatibility of a one- and two-person psychology and the relational school's over-simplified analysis of Freud's awareness of how the individual functions within overlapping and contradictory social and relational matrices. For one thing, as a Darwinian, Freud held that the mind interacts with internal and external environments, that, in fact, the mind is a product of conflicts in and with these environments that are internalized and (partially) repressed by the organism. And even though he did not develop (or know about) Winnicott's concept of the interpersonal transitional space where the object remains undefined between the child and the mother, Freud did develop and place at the center of his work the mechanism of identification which is certainly of the same order, though not the same concept. But, at the same time, Freud worried that the social environment, groups, race, and so on should not become the new intellectual tyranny that squashes the independence and dignity of the individual. Psychoanalysis, therefore, explains how a person develops, how the psychic development of the individual can lead to pathology, and how to repair the pathologies that impede further psychic maturation within a complex interpersonal matrix. And, while it has increased awareness of the mother-child dyad, relational approaches have less to tell us about the ways the unconscious may be death-obsessed than Freud's older dual-drive theory; dual-drive theory has the benefit of having been developed with this question in mind.

More recently, Solms and others have constructed bridges between psychoanalysis and the new brain sciences influencing neuroscience, cognitive psychology, and medicine (in alliance with the drug companies). Solms hopes to substitute Freud's dynamic psychology for cognitive or cybernetic models that are currently in fashion and to link Freud to the contemporary brain research on neurochemical processing. But while the new brain sciences have revolutionized the medical care of certain cognitive deficits, neurochemical imbalances, physical brain traumas, and the dementias, they have very little to tell us at this stage about the role death obsession plays in the unconscious and in the functioning of the neuroses.

The point of this digression into the history of the psychoanalytic movement has been two-fold. It has been undertaken to establish the claim that there has been a relative silence on the subject of the death-obsessed nature of Eros among psychoanalysts. I have tried to show that the idea has either simply not come up or has been demoted from the central problem it became for Freud to a secondary problem of something else (the relation between knowledge and language or between knowledge and subjectivity, for example). Rarely has it been treated as a problem in its own right. Even in Kernberg's work on the instability and aggressiveness of borderline and narcissistic patients, aggression loses its moorings in Freudian drives, becoming a problem in the field of object relations. Spotnitz's important work of mirroring and joining aggression in the transference of narcissistic and schizophrenic patients, too, leaves the nature of aggression unthematized so that some Modern analysts emphasize working with the death drive (Phyllis Meadow) and others do not.[19] This effort to change the subject, moreover, can be placed in context of a political history marked by splits, expulsions, separation, and fragmentation into warring factions which surely can be interpreted as a return of the repressed.

Returning to Freud's focus on the unconscious death obsessions of Eros, however, will be no easy matter in that it takes an act of imagination to think back to the world in which dual-drive theory developed, and I lack the skill to paint the picture that would open that world to my reader's imagination here. Readers may be heartened to know, however, that I provide some background in later chapters, only noting here the importance of taking a second look. I can recommend a second look for many reasons, including the light it sheds on the death obsessions of *our* era, especially our unrelenting destruction of the natural world and its ecosystems while we construct dream worlds of endless youth, credit, and health.[20] Given this, perhaps the fact that dual-drive theory is part of a former *zeitgeist* (this has often been the basis of rejecting it as out of date) may recommend rather than disqualify it as a guide to the perplexed of our age since the alienating effect caused by reading our selves through it may actually free us from some of the unreflective, self-destructive *idées fixes* of our own life-world and allow us some separation from the systems that constitute our contemporary being.

This book examines the proposition that humans are obsessed by death. This death obsession is not a question of existential angst or of a conscious obsession with being dead or dying first and foremost, but it is a matter of the economy of the drives. Quite simply, Eros and Thanatos are locked in perpetual struggle with one another. On the one hand, the death drive seeks to return life to the inorganic world as soon as possible without any delay while, on the other hand, Eros aims to create ever more complicated detours that like a child at play tarries a little before going home (and returning to the inorganic world). This drive conflict underpins the storylines of old television shows like "Wild Kingdom" that followed animals' struggles to live through a drought on the Sierras, for example, dramatizing how the will to survive and adapt to harsh or changing environments lie behind our being living creatures. But, of course, it differs from these "natural" narratives in one crucial respect: the struggle to delay death has in humans come under the sway of language and the Symbolic order so that it is no longer merely "natural." But it has, instead, become a narrative of the symbolic substitution of a loss of the "natural," of a "piece of life" (Lacan calls it libido and *jouissance*) forever cut off which we never stop seeking to rediscover in the desert of the Symbolic (desire).

I want to draw a number of propositions from this premise about dual-drive theory:

First, Eros causes the mind to be as death-obsessed as it is when it is under the influence of the death drive, but Eros causes the mind to be obsessed with delaying or denying death rather than speeding up the organism's return to the inorganic world.

Second, we shall see that Eros is an enormous source of suffering and that the source of this suffering lies in Eros's directing the ego to resist and deny the impulses of the death drives in all its forms. Thus, in *Moses and Monotheism* (1937) Freud argued that the thing that constitutes the Jewish people is not that they were chosen by God or by Moses nor is it that they killed Moses—after all, many peoples have founding or origin myths about the death of a god or a hero who has to be sacrificed (Romulus and Remus is one example, the crucifixion of Christ is another). No, what defines the Jewish people, wrote Freud, is their *forgetting Moses' murder* and the return of the repressed in rituals of prohibition and guilt, while what constitutes Christianity as a community, Freud added, is their (displaced) remembrance of the murder combined with their denial of responsibility or guilt. This act of forgetting, that founds the identity of the Jewish people, in other words, occurs under the sign of a death-denying Eros which pushes the remembrance of the murder (and the mortality) of the hero below the bar of repression.[21] This was also the burning issue when Freud generated a false memory about his childhood so that his pleasure would not be spoiled by guilt while he stood on the Acropolis for the first time and it was what failed a grieving father when he dreamt his son was burning (in reality the son's lifeless body had caught on fire in the next room) as a representation of his own burning guilt and (denied) grief.

Third, this case of the founding of the Jewish people makes the same point as the play "Oedipus Rex" that the more you repress or run from your death drives,[22] the more you run smack into them in the form of a (fantasy of the) *murder of the object*. For Oedipus runs into his father at the crossroads and kills him only after he flees Corinth to defy the oracle that says he will kill his father and sleep with his mother.

Fourth, and this fact leads us to the proposition that the repression of the death drive ends in the return of the repressed—indeed, before death-obsessed Eros murders the object in its imagination *it has already been placed beneath the bar of primary repression*; I say primary repression rather than secondary repression because originally no object is necessary for the drive to be repressed; the drive is so primordial that it is unconscious before it is attached to objects like the mother and father.

Fifth, because death-obsessed Eros is placed beneath the bar of primary repression, it will be maintained and will not be destroyed over time; and because it is maintained as it was in the past, it also serves as the foundation for new elaborations in the present and future when it becomes connected to objects like the mother, father, siblings, bosses, spouses, and enemies. These object relations then become *the object of secondary repression* and the other defenses. The relation between the contents of secondary and primary repression appears in the famous Signorelli gaff discussed by Freud in *The Interpretation of Dreams* when Freud forgets the painter's name after a stranger, whom Freud had engaged in conversation on the train, alludes to the problem of impotence. In sum, the effort to repress or defy the death drive—which defines the aims of death-obsessed Eros—ultimately leads to the forgetting of the apparently unrelated name of the painter that in reality marks the spot of deeper and more disturbing repression.[23]

Sixth, this death-obsessed Eros qua object relations conflicts needs to be elaborated along both the object and the subject axes. It may help to remember that in the relative balance of forces in a person's psyche, it is the influence of Eros on the ego that results in the first projections of internal destructive urges onto objects. The ego would not project the death drives without the influence of Eros because the death drives do not originally seek to cathect objects, and this for two reasons: first, because the death drive is always already under primary repression and second because its original aim is not to destroy objects but to destroy the organism of which they are a part, and it does not need objects to do this. In fact the ego would not push the death drives out to meet objects were it not for the influence of death-obsessed Eros which projects the death drives onto objects to expel them from the interior. In this way, the ego, under the tutelage of Eros, hopes to protect itself by diverting the destructive impulses onto objects and beings in the outside.[24]

Seventh, therefore it is Eros that draws the ego into relations with objects;[25] and Eros—not the death drive—must take responsibility for the original splitting of the ego and world between bad parts which are infested by the death drives and good parts. Apropos this, Kleinian analysts believe (as do the whole object relations community) that welding the two images of the breast into a single image allows the child to repair its perceptions; and Kernberg, for example, maintains that a sense of borderline chaotic emptiness results when the ego cannot bring the good and bad objects together. But we must be careful, for Klein warned us that bringing the good and bad objects together initially causes the infant to become depressed and—this is the point I want to emphasize now—Freud showed throughout his life that ambivalence, which is the consequence of relating to an object as both good and bad, often leads to the ego's envy of the object for having desires and enjoying things independently of its control.

Eighth, for the immature mind, Freud repeatedly argued, will operate as if it is in danger to the degree that the object—especially an object it desires and depends on—remains free of its control and able to independently enjoy itself. In this sense, desire—like wish fulfillment in a dream—seeks to magically guarantee that any outcome with an object is pleasurable (or later profitable) for the subject; and if this is the case with objects of desire, it is equally the case for objects that are the object of the mind's death drives, since the loss of the control of these objects will place the ego in as much or more danger than the loss of the object of desire. This is a perpetual source of worry, Freud saw, for an ego trapped in ambivalent relationships with objects—and if psychoanalysis showed Freud anything it was that all our relationships are more or less ambivalent.

Ninth, thus this ambivalence, Freud noted, draws people into relations that are spoiled by the presence of envy. In fact, envy, Freud added, is present in the negative relations between parent and children during the oedipal complex, which serves as the template for most adult relationships as well. Freud also referred to the envy that binds neighbors (linked to the narcissism of small difference), the envy that unites siblings, the envy of fathers and sons, and more rarely the envy of sons and mothers. Klein, however, stressed that infants already display envy at birth (Augustine said as much sixteen hundred years before) because she saw that envy is a primordial affect—and I would add a primordial affect of death-obsessed Eros turned against objects. Zizek emphasizes that envy "makes me act *against* my own interest" and is a primordial social bond of violence toward one's neighbors.[26] And in *Civilization and Its Discontents*, Freud mentioned that envy is the sort of social bond that unifies people and perennially spoils their happiness, as, for instance, already happens in the *fort/da* game where a fantasy of killing the mother for going away is integral to the game's success in soothing the boy's anxiety of losing his mother.

Tenth, another kind of envy that Freud discussed is penis envy. Much of the early criticism of the idea of penis envy came out of the biological argument that girls are not castrated boys and out of the psychological criticism that women are not morally or psychologically inferior to boys, and, hence, a theory that says women are doomed to see themselves as inferior boys (and inferior to men as creatures of civilization) is monstrous.[27] The first thing that needs to be said about these complaints is that a woman's envy of a man's penis and her fantasy that she had one removed is *fantasy* through and through; it is a little piece of theater staged by and for the pleasure principle to keep the girl from encountering the trauma that she is being treated as less than a boy by her parents and society. Thus, penis envy is to be taken less as a factual statement about women (it obviously is not, and Freud knew it) than an indictment of a society in which girls are made to *envy* an object (the male penis) and turn their death drives against themselves for lacking it. And if there is something outrageous about penis envy, it is not Freud's claim—he is merely the messenger and a sympathetic (albeit imperfect) one at that—but the fact that women are made to see themselves as beings who lack the phallus (from the start) whereas boys are only made to fear that they will never receive it from their father.

Eleventh, girls, then, learn to internalize forms of shame that boys are spared, but formally the envy boys are taught and the envy girls are taught is equivalent. Envy is envy and each gender learns to envy what the other gender enjoys, and the fact that the girl envies a male organ (penis) and the boy envies their father and mother's pleasure is not the relevant point. To the extent that they remain children of envy both genders—male and female—are prone to maintain uncertain and immature forms of subjectivity. And in relation to the subject, that fragile and impermanent "I" that can stand against and try to know the object world, that "I" which Descartes explored and whose existence he hoped to guarantee in the dubious certainty that God would not deceive him as to its being,[28] Freud insisted that the "I" is not constituted by a dishonest genie or an honest god but by its relation to death and the death drive, and from the fact that the subject first emerges in opposition to death.

Twelfth, apropos this recall that Freud created psychoanalysis in part to grieve the death of his father, and its inaugural dreams included "Irma's Injection" which turned on Freud's uncertain identity as doctor and the "You are requested to close the/an eyes" dream that Freud dreamt on the evening of his father's burial service. And what is true about the inauguration of psychoanalysis, Freud wrote, is equally true for the constitution of other subjects. The subject rises through the behest of Eros to defy death, although in reality this heroic image of the subject is an idyll; and just as the dream "You are requested to close the/an eyes" constitutes the subject of analysis in the act of looking away—"closing the/an eyes"—all subjects are forms of looking away or at least looking awry or askance. And from the perspective of the subject, this sideways glancing at the world may literally become a matter of life and death as, for example, it was for the hysterical homosexual patient whom Freud described as having thrown herself in front of a train when her father carelessly tore to shreds her identity—rooted in her sexual revolt—which also was her shield against horror and death.

Thirteenth, but if this is true then it is equally true that Freud did not seek the disintegration of the subject à la the oceanic merging of life and death—but precisely the opposite—he meant to reconstitute the subject, the fragile "I," on the basis of a more mature alliance between the pleasure principle and te reality principle; and thus grounded, the subject would be able to internalize a more *certain reality of death* and the mortality of the subject. Freud, however, was not alone in pursuing this goal. Ferenczi was in basic agreement with Freud on the main points, as we can see by considering his attitude toward a patient who had been molested as a child and whose will to live hung by a string. In her sessions, she would become deeply regressed, childlike, and dependent on Ferenczi who wrote in his clinical notebooks that he counseled (besides greater emotional availability) helping his patient maintain some boundaries against the world. And, rather than giving in to an oceanic merger experience or accepting a total breakdown in regression, as Winnicott seemed to permit his most regressed patients to do, Ferenczi tried to keep the boundaries, and the kissing episodes that so alarmed Freud, when Ferenczi allowed his most regressed patients to hold his hand and kiss him on the head, illustrated the principal of bending so that the analysis did not break.

Fourteenth, *Civilization and Its Discontents* (1930), a book that partially turns on the return of the repressed and the figure of the primal father who defies all limits and knows no boundaries, starts with a denouncement of the oceanic experience; and a careful reading of the book shows that Freud is demonstrating the dangers of Eros freed of all limits. Similarly, anxiety, which is so much on Freud's mind in *Civilization and Its Discontents*, signals the danger that the ego feels when the defenses between life and death drives erected by Eros may be breached.

Fifteen, to illustrate what I mean by this consider a patient of mine who lives in a state of constant panic when I am not physically in his line of sight; even when I am near him, he feels only partially consoled. This poor soul has almost no ability to maintain a boundary between his erotic and destructive impulses and ideas; and as a result he relies on me to keep ideas of death, and the equally alarming thought that he will be unspeakably hurt by someone, from overwhelming him. In other words, I have taken on the role of a parent-guardian in the transference. But I am far from a perfect or ideal object because as a transference object I must be a damaged object, and ultimately

I must not be able to stand up to his persecutory fears. This must be so (at this stage in our analysis) because his fantasy world is organized by a primal image that the phallus has feet of clay; and to the extent that I represent that flawed phallus for him I too must be an imperfect vessel and unable to hold his anxiety well enough. I must remain, in other words, a helpful object but corroded through and through by death,[29] and, therefore, in accord with his transference, unable to help him maintain his boundary defenses when I am away. At such times, he relies on various ritual behaviors to maintain a modicum of control; but Freud explained, in another context, where this may lead: endless prohibitions for keeping the pure and impure apart, cleansing rituals and restrictions, the continuous return of anxiety, and so on. In sum, this patient of mine becomes most anxious and regressed in states bordering on merger experiences where he is unable to effectively use me or his own defenses to manage his death drives.

Sixteenth, Freud already showed us that language is a principal means for addressing the problems created by death-obsessed Eros, and Freud constantly alluded to how verbal play, slips of the pen and tongue, jokes, and so on cover over a trauma and enhance desire. He showed, for instance, how word play often lies behind dream-works, and, as such, how it is vital in masking the latent content of the unconscious by the preconscious wish. The Signorelli gaff has already been mentioned by me as a convenient illustration of forgetting a name to keep an idea of impotence from disturbing Freud's conversation. Forgetting names can also be described as a form of word play in which Signorelli or father must not be recalled because doing so may also arouse repressed thoughts of castration and impotency. Freud also insisted that people not confuse words, images, and drives with each other—each of which are, he wrote, prone to create disturbances of reality in their own registers. Freud, therefore, continuously distinguished between death as a drive (which along with Eros and the pleasure principle, he said, dominates unconscious processes) and death as a word or idea. Thus *Inhibition, Symptom, and Anxiety* (1927) contains long passages where Freud developed the claim that (although it was full of death drives) the word or idea of death cannot appear in the unconscious as a representation of itself because the unconscious cannot signify negations like death or the idea No except when the ideas or words are being *indirectly* and *secondarily* linked to the idea of or word castration—or to some other word or idea that conveys the impression of danger and loss of being. The importance of distinguishing death as a drive and a word reappears in Lacan, who will distinguish between the drive in the Symbolic, Imaginary, and Real. He also will discuss the fact that the unconscious, being structured like a language, is a cauldron of impulses less than it is a register of repressed letters, words, phrases, and narratives joined to various metonyms and metaphors; that is, Lacan wants to make a further distinction than Freud had between the structure of the unconscious—which is of the register of the signifiers—and the register of the drives which is a register of mute repetitions of the compulsions of *jouissance*; and to the extent that we identify Lacan's Real with the world of the drives and trauma than we can also link it to Freud's proposition that the most extreme repetition compulsions verge on an unsayable, and hence largely unmasterable, trauma. In these extreme situations, which Ferenczi was among the first analysts to study in depth, the individual goes on living, but just barely, and without much pleasure, and with the possibility that the ego may simply lose the will to live completely.

Seventeenth, and lastly, while a child may cover over a trauma by throwing a spool of string into the unknown abyss on the other side of a curtain, grown men or women will rely on more intellectually sophisticated symbols and structures to do the same thing. An ancient Western tradition, for example, argues that pursuing the Good is more important than fearing death and a philosopher should love virtue more than fear dying.[30] "The Apology" of Plato provides a famous statement of this view and in the "Theaetetus" Plato has Socrates say that virtuous men "make all haste to escape from the earth to heaven . . . (and so become) like a God as possible." Similarly, in the "Phaedo" Plato has Socrates say that "all who actually engage in philosophy aright are practicing nothing other than dying and being dead," a proposition which Julia Annas tells us refers to a doctrine of "the separation of the soul from the body."[31] What this doctrine expresses about the unconscious, however, is quite simply that the emotional need to disavow the mind's obsession with death goes on at the highest regions of cultural output.

The Romantic, too, is obsessed by the proximity of love and death. In this, Romantic love calls to mind (the very different case of) the doctor who gives his patient six more months to live when he does not pay his bill, for the Romantic must never reach his or her destination—which is death, and to keep death from arriving, the ego, in the name of Eros, draws on a store of images and fantasies that all turn on representations of delay or deferment.[32] The Romantic has to keep everything in a state of suspension and tension so that the clock never strikes midnight. Recall Freud's discussion in *Beyond the Pleasure Principle* of Plato's "Symposium." Mankind, Freud quoted the poet saying, was once whole until an angry Zeus cut them in two so that human beings are now and forever incomplete and unhappy, finding happiness only when they fall into the arms of their other half. But notice: I have not mentioned Eros as the protector of life, and the poet says quite the opposite. He says that romantic union brings bliss *and* the descent to death. Eros seems to be a God with more than one thing on his mind. On the one hand, he hopes to make one where there are two and, therefore, to be a therapeutic God who repairs the damage done by Zeus. But, on the other hand, he is the herald of death and warns his devotees to beware of what they desire, counseling delay, and advising them to be satisfied with their longings; this is the Eros Freud has in mind when he mentions that Eros seeks to delay death and so serve life.

We can track this romantic ideal to many literary parryings (twins, doppelgangers) starting with Adam and Eve and including Sherlock Holmes and Moriarty, and the myth of Narcissus falling into his watery image and drowning (in another version he is transformed into the flower while staring into his reflection).[33] The messages of these stories are all the same: the individual must never meet his twin, except in a deadly embrace. The same message appears in Gothic horror tales, and *Frankenstein* is certainly a variation on this theme.

The same prohibition also structures the movie *The Third Man* (1949). Made in the later 1940s, starring Orson Wells, the film is shot in postwar Vienna, a city divided into occupational zones controlled by the British, French, Americans, and Russians. Taking place in the period before the economic miracle began, Vienna is a bombed out and ruined city whose citizens are dehumanized and forced to scrounge around to exist. The plot begins when Holly Martins comes to Vienna because Harry had offered him a job and then later to find out about his old pal Harry Lime, who is supposed to be dead but turns out to be very much alive. Harry has been running a smuggling ring and distributing watered-down penicillin to hospitals. After many children died, he faked his death to get the authorities off his trail, but Holly's nosing around will lead to his discovery.

The conventions of Romance that I mentioned above explain why Holly only meets Harry four times in the movie. He sees him hiding in the shadows once. Once, they meet on the famous Ferris wheel in the Prater. They meet again at the cafe, when Harry escapes into the sewers. And they meet when Holly kills Harry in the sewers. In other words, Harry and Holly just miss each other three times, causing the suspense to rise like in a Beethoven symphony before reaching its resolution. For, far more than Anna, it is Holly who functions as the other half of Harry in the film, and for this reason it is possible to interpret the film as a miniature *A Thousand and One Nights* in which the game is to bring Holly ever closer to Harry without having them truly meet; that is, the game is to keep them from reaching the end, which will be the death of Harry. Thus, something always comes between Harry and Holly, call it a lack of understanding, especially on Holly's part, that keeps the real basis of their friendship under repression, but which is, for that reason, most propitious for all concerned since it allows the story to go on.

The story turns on Holly's disillusionment, which parallels an analysis (but the end is quite different). Thus, the first three meetings between Holly and Harry (one accidental, the others planned) in the divided city of Vienna follow this progression: a. Holly accidentally sees a dead man; b. Harry is now very real, but is more of a stranger to Holly; c. the ideal image of Harry is shattered and Holly contemplates betraying Harry. It takes the entire film before Holly decides his (Imaginary) destiny consists in fulfilling Harry's desire to die rather than be captured like a rat (Harry might say to not die like the suckers); and, if we judge them by their end, Holly's association with Harry has been a long preparation for this encounter at the crossroads to Thebes.

Among the multiple ironies in play at this moment in the film is that Holly becomes a mirror image of Harry, who has maimed and murdered hundreds of people by distributing watered-down penicillin on the black market, when he finally kills Harry; even if Holly murders for love and pity and Harry for pleasure and profit, Holly and Harry become (if only in that instant), when Holly shoots Harry, One; and this great Romantic epiphany may be the only moment in Holly's relationship with Harry that is not based on a pack of lies and falsehoods (although Holly is in other instances *no Harry*, as Anna lets him know in no uncertain terms).

And then there is Anna. Perhaps more than anyone, except Major Calloway, the British military policeman who is trying to capture Harry and protect Anna, certainly more than Holly when he arrives in Vienna, Anna's image of Harry is nearer the real Harry, and yet she vehemently denies the case being built by Calloway because she is the good hysteric in the way Lacan defines hysteria in *Seminar* XVIII. She wants to expose Harry at the same time as she wants to protect him, and her ambivalence ties her up in knots. Ironically, she martyrs herself to an idealized image of him that in her heart of hearts she knows is false because Harry has become her Imaginary life line, her anchor against death and despair. Did Harry not save her when the hounds were threatening by getting her forged papers, and would he not save her again if he could? Indeed, her self-delusions extend to Holly and herself too, and so, ironically, she kicks Holly while he is down (this being the equivalent to an erotic murder) in the famous scene with the rows of linden trees following Harry's funeral when she walks past him as if he was not there (so, she too became a mirror image of the death-dealing Harry in the end) and whose solidarity with Harry she cannot accept.

Indeed, Harry's ghost hovers over the film long before the penultimate scene following Harry's funeral. In one respect, he is like the ghost of Hamlet's father, but instead of demanding revenge from a lackluster son, Harry (while alive) makes ghostly demands on Anna and Holly. As we saw, he demands Holly should be the one to kill him. What he demands from Anna is something more complicated. He wants that she should desire a dead man; and, in fact, even after she knows Harry is still alive she memorializes him like some fallen hero, and even when everyone can see that it was Harry who betrayed her to the Russians she cannot, because she cannot change her image of Harry which has to remain like granite—unaffected by facts or by the passage of time.

To conclude, there once were Sphinxes marking the graves of children all over the ancient world. And although they only remain as objects of curiosity and beauty in museums today, in a very real sense we all continue to erect monuments to mark and to divert our attentions from our own unconscious grief, or to symbolically show that we have conquered death and found the way out of the labyrinth of death and despair.

We mortal creatures need to escape the trauma of existence into the pleasure principle. We need to be able to negate reality, to replace unpleasure with fantasy, substitute painful reality with magical thinking; in short, we need to have the gift of misreading painful situations sometimes. Such distortions of reality are necessary for life[34] and the aesthetic experience; however, as any Darwinian knows—and Freud was a Darwinian—the ability to make realistic assessments of one's environment and determine when and to what degree one is in danger is vital to survival. Life would not be worth much if people reacted to a hungry lion as if it were a pussy cat,[35] and a person can—people regularly do—rely too much on such flights from reality.

One result of analysis is that it helps people to enjoy more (à la the pleasure principle) and to bond to others better (à la Eros), but without compromising the reality principle too severely. It brings Eros and the pleasure principle into a better and more harmonious alliance with the love of truth, a love which cannot be separated from the development of the whole person. Unfortunately, from the start of life, the love of reality is not as important for survival as expelling the death drives. Children do not have to tolerate much reality because they have the protection of their parents and the adult world, and so they feel only limited pressure to limit their pleasure (until their infantile sexual fantasies come tumbling down on their heads and they are forced to admit more reality—although this reality will be wrapped in a new layer of fantasies as well); and, yet, they are under immediate and constant pressure to expel or sublimate their death drives and to protect themselves from the destructive force in others; and, therefore, they are drawn into relations of dependency and envy with others from the start of life, and they have to learn the value of the love of truth only gradually as they mature. Psychoanalysts, then, must help people to accept limits to their desires and fears (and I am about to say help the subject through love).[36]

Freud's life-long obsession with the date of his death and his fainting episodes underscore the fact that death-obsessed Eros is a sore spot in his unconscious, as is his continued insistence, throughout his life, that the unconscious cannot represent death in itself; for, while this idea makes sense while Freud adheres to libido theory it becomes untenable once he claims the two fundamental drives in the unconscious are a life and a death drive. Adhering to a distinction between death as a drive (that is functioning in the unconscious) and death as a representation (that can only appear in the unconscious as a signifier in a chain of signifiers that ultimately goes back to the root signifier "castration") does not really make sense anymore, especially given Freud's own illumination of the destructive fantasies.[37]

In the coming chapters, readers will gain a better appreciation of the fears and anxieties that arise from death-obsessed Eros in the minds of residents and staff working in nursing homes as well as in the transference and counter-transferences between these two groups, but, first, I want to explore death obsession as a theme in the works of psychoanalysts such as Freud, Lacan, and Klein in greater detail.

NOTES

1. Carrying out a phenomenological reduction also did not interest me since my work as an analyst turns on the irreducibility of an unconscious structure that resists such generalizations. For an effort to create just such a phenomenological reduction of the unconscious of specific patients see Gerhard Fichtner, ed., *Sigmund Freud-Ludwig Binswanger Correspondence, 1908–1938* (New York: The Other Press, 2003). In a different manner, Lacan attempted to do what many others were attempting in the twentieth century: to explore the limits to creating a science of subjectivity. See Francois Roustang, *The Lacanian Delusion*, trans. Gregg Sims (Oxford: Oxford University Press, 1980) for an illuminating if hostile critique of these pretensions.
2. Martin Bergman, ed., *The Hartmann Era* (New York: The Other Press, 2000).
3. Rollo May and other American analysts presented a far more optimistic existentialism than was developed in Europe. See Rollo May, *The Discovery of Being: Writings in Existential Psychology* (New York: W. W. Norton & Co., 1994).
4. The dominance of logical positivism after World War II (despite challenges from Marxism and Existentialism) may be a related fact.
5. The anti-ideology movement of the fifties was the result. Ostensibly a call to scientific neutrality and a criticism of the ideologically driven politics of the inter-war years, it was really an attack on Marxism by the Right. Similarly, after the collapse of the Soviet Union, the end of history discourse was coupled to a new end of ideology discourse which again meant an end to Marxist discourses.
6. Russell Jacoby, *Social Amnesia: A Critique of Contemporary Psychology* (New York: Transaction Publication, 1997).

7. Marcuse saw its production as potentially revolutionary. Zizek, however, sees it as the essence of the superego command to enjoy! in consumer culture. Compare Herbert Marcuse, *Eros and Civilization: A Philosophical Inquiry in Freud* (New York: Beacon Press, 1955) and Slavoj Zizek, *Violence: Big Ideas/Small Books* (New York: Picador, 2008).

8. Compare their revolutionary optimism with the pessimism Adorno conveyed in his famous statement that no one can write poetry after Auschwitz—as if the imagination collapsed in the face of so much barbarism à la Beckett's prose.

9. Like many film theorists who misread Lacan, many feminists in America often misunderstand him and what he had to say about female desire and everyone's desire for the mother.

10. Carolyn Burke, Naomi Schor, Margaret Whitford, eds., *Engaging with Irigaray* (New York: Columbia University Press, 1994).

11. There is a disturbing conflation (unanalyzed) between a fleeting and contingent "feminine *jouissance*" and a *jouissance* of death; that is a complex conflating of a mode of *jouissance* that Lacan insists "does not exist but is still in the realm of the possible (feminine *jouissance*) an "impossible" because forbidden *jouissance* of death that the Symbolic order has come to replace: that the Symbolic exists by making the *jouissance* of death "impossible." But what the exact relation between this "impossible" mode of being and this other "possible and contingent" one is remains unanalyzed. Such analysis requires going deeper into the relation between the possible modes of *jouissance* and sexuality, on the one hand, and the *jouissance* or seduction of death, on the other hand. A starting place may be a dialogue opening between Bataille's reader and the readers of Lacan and Irigaray.

12. Andre Breton liked to equate the "marvelous" with states of "intoxication" and, like the Romantics had before, with the shattering or death of the subject. See Surrealism's interest in occultism and the link there between spiritualism and eroticism. See Andre Breton, *Manifeste surréaliste*, 1924, and Andre Breton, André Masson, Joan Mirro, and Salvador Dali, *André Breton: Surrealism and Painting* (New York: MFA Publications, 2002). It has to be said too that many Lacanians (the ones who adhere to the later Lacan's turn to the problem of feminine sexuality and *jouissance* in general) are also attracted by the idea of a fleeting transgression of Symbolic that looks an awful lot like a postmodern form of erotic-materialist mysticism (à la Bataille).

13. Roland Barthes, *The Semiotic Challenge*, trans. Richard Howard (New York: Hill and Wang, 1988).

14. Roustang, *The Lacanian Delusion*, 32.

15. Judith Butler and Joan Scott, eds., *Feminists Theorize the Political* (New York: Routledge, 1992) and Sara Salih and Judith Butler, *The Judith Butler Reader* (Malden, Mass.: Blackwell Pub., 2004).

16. Differences rooted in culture have appeared in the literature more slowly but they have begun to appear nevertheless.

17. It reflects nostalgia for the mother (in an age when mothers have taken on new social roles alongside motherhood).

18. Christopher Lasch, *The Culture of Narcissism: American Life in an Age of Diminishing Expectations* (New York: W. W. Norton & Co., 1978; 1991).

19. Hyman Spotnitz, *Modern Psychoanalysis of the Schizophrenic Patient: Theory of the Technique* (New York: Grune & Stratton, 2004); Spotnitz and Phyllis W. Meadow, *Treatment of the Narcissistic Neuroses* (New York: Manhattan Center for Advanced Psychoanalytic Studies, 1995); Phyllis W. Meadow and Charles Lemert, *The New Psychoanalysis* (Lanham, Md.: Rowman & Littlefield, 2003).

20. The student revolts of the sixties already began to challenge the view that prosperity will lead to happiness and global security. We can also note that in the 1920s, especially in war-ravaged central and Eastern Europe, things looked different, and the dual-drive theory is in part an artifact of that different time and place, in particular, its pessimism about the future. On the replacement of the concept of nature by the simulacra, see Jean Baudrillard, *Simulacra and Simulation*, trans. Shiela Faria Glaser (Ann Arbor: University of Michigan Press, 1995); Baudrillard, *Simulations* (New York, Semiotext(e), Inc., 1983).

21. In other cases—and this may partially be the secret of Christian anti-Semitism—the destruction of the object is displaced onto a proxy.

22. The difference is that in the one story (that of the founding of the Jewish people), the murdered object is Moses—the founder of a people—while in the Oedipal story, the murdered object is Oedipus' biological father—the founder of Oedipus the man.

23. Thus, as I just said, the death obsessions of Eros will cause endless suffering and anxiety in the family, among friends, in the world, and so on; and, this suffering will cause the ego to react by the only means it has at its disposal: it will respond with defenses, fixations, secondary repression, and sublimation. Analysts who regularly focus on the conflicts surrounding what I call the secondary repression of death-obsessed Eros, the problems that develop around object relations, self psychology, relational dynamics, and so on, must remain sensitive to how these secondary conflicts develop from drive conflicts that remain under primary repression.

24. Very soon, Eros will need to protect the organism (and this includes the breast that provides food, warmth, and love—that is, which is the prosthesis that keeps life alive) from the return of the death drives—now seen to be coming from the enraged or poisonous object.

25. The death drive originally performs a purely passive role in allowing its transfer onto objects.

26. Zizek, *Violence*, 2006.

27. Freud speculated that while boys learn to fear losing the phallus, girls are taught to internalize the idea that they are inferior boys because they (for some reason) do not have a penis.

28. Einstein, in a different context, thought god does not play dice with the universe.

29. This is one reason why divine beings that live outside of time are invented.

30. This can be read as intellectualizations and reaction formations against the death-obsessed Eros that constitutes the subject.

31. Julia Annas, *Platonic Ethics, Old and New* (Cornell, N.Y.: Cornell University Press, 2000), 60–61.

32. We will see that Lacan, and in a more explicit way Alain Miller, Zizek, and other later Lacanians, will criticize the lure of the ideal of a lost wholeness and the ideal of the One which originates in the Imaginary register created when we looked into the mirror and see a vision of our totality reflected in our mother's gaze. This Imaginary is, therefore, a cause and a byproduct of desire. The quest for being in the One, then, is a lure.

33. The myth warns against becoming too self-absorbed with one's own image.

34. Friedrich Nietzsche, *The Nietzsche Reader* (New York: Wiley-Blackwell, 2006).

35. Or, if they fantasized that pulling out a thorn would turn the frightening lion into a pussy cat.

36. At least I hope to show that only love of the truth will give the ego sufficient strength to neutralize the death drives and overcome the ancient paths of dealing with them. The more compromises the ego makes, the more it can come under the influence of the death drive—except when it learns to sublimate the drives to love of truth and neutralizes rather than masks them behind the pursuit of pleasure and Eros.

37. This resistance to facing the death obsessed nature of Eros in the unconscious must have played a part in Freud's poor judgments before and during the *Anschluss*. For, Freud seems to almost have been paralyzed when it came to facing the Nazi danger. This paralysis can be seen in his never really doing anything to get himself, his family, or friends out of Austria until it is almost too late and he really had to depend on the intercessions of Jones, Bonaparte, and Bullock to make his narrow escape to "die in freedom." Freud's own explanation that he was too old to think of leaving the city he loved and hated does not really make sense since he made no plans to get his family out ahead of time either, even though Ferenczi and others pleaded with him to leave as early as 1933, and even though Freud warns others, including Stephan Zweig, and the whole Berlin society to get out of Germany. And, if Freud had so much difficulty facing the death drive and reacting intelligently to it, we hardly can expect others to do better.

2

What Is a Death Wish in Early Freud?

The worst was this; my love was my decay.

—Shakespeare, "Sonnet 80"

Freud's early writings describe unconscious death wishes. But these death wishes are presented by Freud as the byproducts of children's psychosexual conflicts with other family members, and as the byproducts of extremely hypocritical demands that society and the family impose on the individual to repress their sexuality and to compel their acceptance of the norms of the Symbolic order. In other words, death is not treated by Freud as a drive yet, but, instead, death is only seen to be a representation of a wish to remove an object inhibiting the fulfillment of an erotic wish. We, however, can draw two conclusions from this original position on what a death wish is. First, at this time the emergence of a death wish is tied to the appearance of a dangerous object that has the power (or is thought to have the power) to inhibit a libidinal satisfaction. Second, the role of the death wish is to clear away the impediment to libidinal satisfaction, and as such it is connected to the pleasure principle and to the fulfillment of an erotic wish. Apropos this, Freud stresses at this time that the principle form that a repressed death wish from childhood takes is the wish to make some offending object "go away," to leave the field unobstructed so that the child's libido can flow unimpeded to its object free of hindrance or anxiety.

One can think of a death wish, then, as a second order wish, something that helps make the fulfillment of an erotic wish possible. Thus, children may wish that daddy will go away or not return home or that a sibling may fly away and not return anymore, but these wishes are, at least originally, innocent and they mean little more than I want what I want. It goes without saying that Freud stresses that these wishes to get rid of someone are only one side of an ambivalent conflict, so that the wish to make daddy go away will always be opposed by other loving wishes to be like daddy and by wishes to make the whole knotty situation go away by becoming unconscious or preconscious. Freud also says, when speaking of childhood death wishes, that the impulse to repress the death wish is especially pronounced during and after the oedipal complex and during and after puberty. The case of "Little Hans" exemplifies how a death wish can be integral to the formation of a symptom once it undergoes repression—specifically, the "Little Hans" case illustrates one way that a wish to get rid of daddy can be transformed into a complex animal phobia with irrational fears of biting horses and of horses that fall down.

In this respect, the wish to make someone die occupies an in-between space in Freud's writing at this time that is also, paradoxically, the space of concepts like anxiety, which, like death, will be given a whole new significance in Freud's second drive theory after 1920. Thus, Freud's early theory of anxiety contains the notion that pent up anxiety causes many forms of neurotic behavior because pent up anxiety is itself a symptom of sexual repression. In reaching this conclusion, Freud draws on the work of many contemporary sexologists like Havelock Ellis and the psychiatric research of men like Emile Charcot with hysterics, all of which leads Freud to conclude that anxiety is an affective state caused when pent up libido is somehow transformed into a state of nervousness, even though Freud cannot say how this transformation from libido to anxiety occurs. Moreover, Freud realizes that anxiety is not a single type of affect, but, rather, that anxiety can be produced by a variety of disturbances, including organic disturbances, psychosexual disturbances caused by too much sexual repression in society, and psychosexual disturbances caused by other sexual and psychological conflicts in families. He also believes that many anxiety disorders originate from the reproduction during adulthood of infantile libidinal conflicts; these are the so-called transference neuroses, and they can be distinguished from the actual neuroses which do not have a source in childhood.

Whatever the source of an anxiety may be, however, Freud at this time treats anxiety as a nervous condition caused by the mysterious conversion of pent up libido into a state of nervous tension and energy in the body. Anxiety, then, is also a second order concept, and, like death wishes, it is caused by the repression of libido.[1] Or, to say this differently, at this time Freud believes that both anxiety and the death wish are symptoms of sexual repression. Death wishes, however, cannot be equated with anxiety if for no other reason than that they are not an affective state like anxiety. But mental representations of a wish to get rid of an impediment to the satisfaction of an erotic wish, Freud already knows, are often accompanied by states of anxiety and guilt. One can, of course, imagine situations where someone has a death wish without anxiety, or that someone has anxiety that is not accompanied by a death wish, but there is an obvious connection between the two in Freud's mind. But, whether the death wish arises as a cause or as an effect of the conversion of pent up libido into anxiety or guilt is largely situational in that anxiety may function as a source of a death wish (say, for example, when castration anxiety leads the child to fantasize the father will go away) or as its consequence. The appearance of guilt in the field of representations, then, reflects a higher level of conflict in which the wish to remove an obstacle to satisfaction elicits guilt and feelings of remorse. Freud is now coming to see that guilt often operates as the primary link between the death wish and anxiety.

Perhaps some readers may have asked themselves why I am focusing on death wishes when the commentaries on Freud's work, especially commentaries on his early pre-1920 writings, rarely mention them. But, in response, I would wonder at the relative silence in the literature on this topic, given the fact that Freud feels that the death wish, the wish to remove an obstruction to an erotic pleasure, is so important to a theory of the wish and to a theory of desire, judging solely from the frequency with which Freud mentions people who are sickened by some repressed death wish in works like *The Interpretation of Dreams* (1900). One may even be tempted to say that the death wish is, for Freud, one of the classic examples of a wish that, in time, either when the wish is formed or later in puberty, becomes an object of repression and anxiety itself. One, for example, can read the conflicts raging around the oedipal complex in this way as narratives about the desire to remove the father opposing other desires to identify with the father as a model for the ego.

It will take another twenty years, however, before Freud treats death as a drive as well as a representation. And, therefore, this chapter will focus on Freud's first and only position for over twenty years, that is, his position that death wishes are wishes or kinds of desires. However, rather than just repeat Freud's changing positions on the question of what a death wish is, I want to do something a little more ambitious. I want to interpret how Freud's own death wishes, as revealed in his analysis of two dreams, affect his thought processes, and, finally, how Freud's own way of thinking about death prepares him to make the leap from the idea that death wishes are only wishes to the idea that they are representations of a conflict between a death drive and Eros. For, even when Freud maintains that a death wish is only a representation, and not a drive, he presents increasingly nuanced descriptions of death wishes. And, he comes to increasingly differentiate the death wishes of different sorts of people: including hysterics, people with anxiety neuroses, people with narcissistic disorders, and so on.

But let us begin by returning to the 1890s, to a time when Freud has a number of dreams that will eventually find their way into *The Interpretation of Dreams* (1900), that is, to a time before Freud conceives of death as a drive. To make my point, I will select two dreams. The first specimen dream occurs around 1897, and, according to Freud, develops into the following narrative:

> I am going into a kitchen for a pudding. Three women are standing there, one of whom is the landlady, and she is turning something in her hand as though making dumpling (*Knodel*). She answers that I must wait until she is finished (not clearly as speech). I grow impatient and go away offended. I put on an overcoat: but the first one I try is too long for me. I take it off again, rather surprised that it is trimmed with fur. A second coat that I put on has a long stripe with Turkish markings on it. A stranger with a long face and a short pointed beard comes up and prevents me from putting it on, declaring it is his. Then I show him that it is covered all over with Turkish embroidery. He asks: "What are the Turkish (markings, stripes . . .) to you?" But then we are quite friendly with one another.[2]

Although Freud only stresses the oedipal complex in the 1900s, the oedipal nature of the dream should be apparent, with the fur-trimmed coat signifying the women's genitals and the long Turkish markings on the coat that the stranger prevents him from putting on signifying the same. But, death wishes are plentiful, but repressed, in this dream too. And, it is these death wishes that I want to highlight so that we can begin to make out where, and in what ways, death wishes function in Freud's unconscious at this time.

To find the death wishes in the dream, however, requires linking elements of the manifest dream to latent dream thoughts about Freud's frustrated unconscious erotic wishes for his mother. This will include a discussion of Freud's fear of being pushed out of the maternal orbit by a younger rival; that is, a fear that Freud is being neglected by his mother, who is lavishing her attention on a rival—a fear, I may add, that Freud turns from a passive fear of neglect and abandonment into an active decision to leave at the end of the dream, but which, for all that, cannot mask the primal association with neglect and with being cast out of Eden (the kitchen) into the cold (hence, the allusions to coats), adult world, either.

We can flush the death wishes out of their hiding places in the dream by looking more closely at what the dream says. In particular, the dream begins in the kitchen, where the dreamer goes to get some pudding, and where

Freud sees the three women. One, the landlady, tells him (in garbled speech) to wait while she makes something like a dumpling. Annoyed, he leaves. In this scene, then, the dreamer returns to a time and place (the kitchen) where women dominate his unconscious oral fantasies.[3] One can surmise that the kitchen represents some kind of very early ideal for the dreamer, in the same manner that Otto Rank later idealizes the mother's womb, but such a conclusion would be too hasty. For this womb or early post-natal world (if that is what it is) is far from the sort of untroubled space that Rank imagines prenatal life to have been. Freud lets us know this in his associations to the dream, where he tells us that the three women remind him of *the three Fates* of Greek mythology that Shakespeare names the weird sisters in *Macbeth.* Furthermore, the three Fates, as well as the scene of the landlady rolling a *knodel* between her hands, reminds Freud of a boyhood memory of watching his mother roll her fingers together until she produces a clump of dirt and epidermis to illustrate to her astonished son that everyone comes from and returns to the earth:

> When I was six years old and was given my first lessons by my mother, I was expected to believe that we were all made of earth and must therefore return to earth. This did not suit me and I expressed doubts of the doctrine. My mother thereupon rubbed the palms of her hands together—just as she did making dumplings, except that there was no dough between them—and she showed me the blackish scales of epidermis produced by the friction as proof that we were made of earth. My astonishment at this ocular demonstration knew no bounds and I acquiesced in the belief I was later to hear expressed in the words: "Thou owe Nature a death."

The associations to the dream, then, extend back to a nodal concern with the sovereign nature of life and death. And, the orally frustrating landlady signifies the place of the mother in Freud's unconscious transformed into a goddess of birth, fate, and death, a mother-Fate (Mother Earth) who holds men's fortunes in her hands and, therefore, elicits fear and devotion from them.

This suggests that, even at this young age, the place of the mother in Freud's unconscious is full of erotic wishes and death wishes that depict the mother as the angel of life and death, that is, the dream suggests, even as a boy, that the place of the mother is a nodal point of erotic wishes and death wishes in Freud's unconscious. I do not mean to suggest that when Freud reports this dream he sees all these connections between his own childish erotic wishes and death wishes, on the one hand, and the world of maternal images, on the other hand. He obviously does not. And, in the coming decade, his theorizing will focus more on the central role that the oedipal triangle plays in the formation of the neuroses than it will focus on the role of the place of the mother in the unconscious as a site of clashing erotic wishes and death drives. And, yet, we can see that Freud, without noticing what he has done, has touched on the deep psychological link between the place of the mother and the most primal impulses toward life and death that, genetically speaking at least, precedes the formation of the place of the father in the unconscious as a site of contestation between erotic wishes, death wishes, and castration anxiety.

Indeed, what is striking about Freud's interpretation of dreams like this one is his tendency (dramatized so nicely in this dream) to move on from exploring the place of the mother in the unconscious as a site of erotic wishes and death wishes to the place of the father in the oedipal complex too quickly. Not that the father complex is any less important than Freud thinks it is (although many analysts today think it is not of any importance at all), but that Freud seems less willing to explore the place of the mother in his unconscious with the same tenacity that he investigates the place of the father. Apropos this, Freud will make two statements at different moments that deserve to be juxtaposed with one another. In the first, Freud famously writes that nothing is more significant in a man's life than the loss of his father and, in the second, he writes that a boy's relation with his mother is the least ambivalent relation a man has in his life, but his dreams, of course, suggest otherwise.[4] And, according to Sophie Freud, Freud returned from his weekly visits to his mother with an upset stomach.[5]

We can see that Freud's eroticized death wishes are tied to his childhood images of his mother in another part of the dream where a rival for her affection appears. This rival, however, does not appear as himself in the manifest dream, but in the form of a *knodel*, for, Freud reports that he feels displeasure when the inn-hostess-mother makes something that *resembles a knodel*—something, Freud is quick to add, that also is "a living creature." The *knodel*, then, is both a dumpling and "a living creature" and, we can surmise that this dumpling-living creature may also symbolize a baby feeding at its mother's breast, for Freud adds in the association phase: "I knew that one of the three women—the inn-hostess in the dream—was the *mother who gives life*, and furthermore—as in my own case—*gives the living creature its first nourishment*. Love and hunger, I reflected, meet at a woman's breast."

These feelings of libidinal frustration are associated with the place of the mother in Freud's unconscious where the landlady is "turning something in her hand as though making dumplings," that is, where the inn-hostess is making a *knodel-baby*; and this leads to a death wish that the baby would die and go away, a death wish that Freud understands to be the expression of a wish to remove an obstacle to an erotic satisfaction (the pudding) just as Freud relates a patient of his wish in childhood that "a flock of children, all her brothers, sisters, and cousins, were romping in a meadow. Suddenly they grew wings, flew up in the air, and were gone."[6]

That this *knodel* is Julius, Freud's younger brother who died after one and a half years of life, is made obvious by other associations to the dream, including the allusion to "owe Nature a death" mentioned in regards to his mother's dirty hands, for, as Freud explains in his commentary on the now famous "Non Vixit" dream, he wished Julius to "go away and not return" as a child.[7] This association to a death wish reminds Freud that, as a young boy, he seemed to have murdered Julius by wishing him dead.

We have here, then, a psychical complex in which a death wish that is supposed to remove an inhibition to satisfaction of an erotic wish has aroused profound guilt feelings of remorse. One can say that this remorse is both misplaced because the wish is not the cause of Julius's death and the beginning of Freud's sense of morality which Freud says is ground in remorse and guilt. But, at the same time, we also can say that the death wish is subject to being forgotten (but not gone) so that it has to be remembered as a dream. Indeed, Julius, the main subject of the dream, gets unceremoniously replaced by a *knodel*, while the death wish itself appears as a frustrated desire to leave the kitchen.

All things considered, then, the need to deny the death wish is stronger in this dream than the wish to distort the frustrated erotic desire for the mother. Leaving the kitchen, however, may screen other distressing oral anxieties connected to a form of depression. For the Freud biographer Louis Breger suggests that Freud's mother may have become "unavailable in her unhappy state following" Julius's death, which quickly follows on the heels of the death of Amalia's brother Julius, his namesake. The dream, therefore, may revitalize old, buried memories of losing his mother to a rival and of losing her to her own emotional unavailability and depression when the two Juliuses die. And, if we accept Lacan's claim that losing the mother is sometimes connected to a fear that the subject will die without the mother's presence, Freud's guilt may also have stirred up unconscious death anxieties, too; a conclusion that Freud's own work supports when he discusses the connections between depression and the loss of the object in "Mourning and Melancholia" (1917).

Moreover, the fact that "Mourning and Melancholia" also is a study of the narcissistic disorders strongly suggests an association exists between anxieties that the subject will be abandoned and die, certain death wishes, and certain narcissistic disorders based on the loss of the object. Apropos all of what we have been saying, in "Female Sexuality" (1931), Freud will write these sadly poignant lines:

> The turning away from the mother is accompanied by hostility; the attachment to the mother ends in hate. . . . The reproach against the mother which goes back furthest is that she gave the child too little milk—which is construed against her as a lack of love. The next accusation against the child's mother flares up when the next baby appears in the nursery. If possible the connection with oral frustration is preserved: the mother could not or would not give the child anymore milk because she needed the nourishment for the new arrival. In cases in which the two children are so close in age that lactation is prejudiced by the second pregnancy, this reproach acquires a real basis, and it is a remarkable fact that a child, even with an age difference of only eleven months, is not too young to take notice of what is happening. But what the child grudges the unwanted intruder and rival is not only the suckling but all the other signs of maternal care. It feels that it has been dethroned, despoiled, damaged in its rights; it casts a jealous hatred upon the new baby and develops a grievance against the faithless mother.[8]

The connections between erotic frustration and hidden death wishes, however, are not exhausted by the place of the mother as a site of opposing erotic wishes and death wishes in the unconscious in this dream. And, it is possible to excavate an entirely different level of erotic wishes and death wishes that linked to Freud's adult life, and to the place death occupies in it. Included in this level of excavation are numerous erotic wishes and death wishes clustered around the ideas-words "addiction" and "cigars." Cigars are on Freud's mind at the time of the dream, and these associations are often accompanied by powerful, and powerfully frustrated, unconscious erotic wishes and feelings, too. For, in 1895 Freud learns from Josef Breuer that he (Freud) has a heart condition—and Freud writes to Wilhelm Fliess that he now is convinced that he will suffer a fatal heart aneurism in four or five years.[9] Fliess responds to Freud's letter by telling Freud to give up his cigars, something Freud fails to do on a number of occasions. These conflicts appear in the form of an unconscious *knodel*-cigar in the dream, which is the focal point for many erotic wishes and death wishes, expressed thematically in "Sexuality and the Aetiology of the Neuroses" (1898) where Freud writes that "narcotics are meant to serve directly or indirectly as a substitute for the lack of sexual satisfaction";[10] and, all these frustrated desires stir up Freud's anxiety about dying, specifically his superstition that he will die either at fifty-one or at sixty-two years old and it also stirs up unconscious associations to Ernst Fleischl von Marxow—a man whom Freud calls an ideal, and who dies from a cocaine overdose that Freud prescribes to him in 1891 to help wean him off of a morphine addiction,[11] that is, beginning from the simple definition of the death wish as a desire to remove an obstruction to an erotic wish, we have arrived at a case where the satisfaction of an erotic desire has become synonymous with Freud's own death in his unconscious, and, more generally, we have arrived at a situation where the satisfaction of an addiction is associated with the death of a friend and a fear of his own premature demise.

If the preceding dream highlights the often-overlooked connection between the place of the mother and a cluster of erotic wishes and death wishes in Freud's unconscious, the next dream I want to discuss, also from *The Interpretation of Dreams*, will highlight the place of the father, or to be more precise, it will highlight some of the erotic wishes and death wishes that converge around Freud's unconscious desire to assume the Symbolic function within his own family. As such, this dream can be compared with other episodes in Freud's life fruitfully, such as the famous episodes when Freud faints (usually in the presence of Jung), for, these fainting episodes carry the Symbolic meaning of dying, or of being overcome (swooning) by the erotic demands of the Other, especially since these fainting episodes touch on not only Freud's unconscious desire to assume the symbolic function, but they also touch on his wish to name his successor and to designate the time and form of succession.

Such interesting comparisons, however, will have to wait for a latter date since they would take us too far from our present topic, which is a dream in which Freud's wish to assume the Symbolic function attracts a number of erotic and death wishes. The dream goes as follows:

> A palace on the sea. Later it does not lie directly on the edge of the sea, but on a narrow canal leading into the sea. A certain Herr P is the governor. I am standing with him in a great reception room with three windows, and in front of them projecting walls rise like castle battlements. I have been assigned to the occupying force, perhaps as a volunteer naval officer. We are afraid of the immanent arrival of enemy warships, as we are in a state of war. Herr P intends to leave; he gives me instructions about what is to be done if what we fear does happen. His ailing wife is with the children in the vulnerable palace. When the bombardment begins, the great hall is to be cleared. He is breathing heavily and makes to go away; I detain him; and ask how I can get news to him if necessary. He says something in reply, *but then immediately falls down dead.* I have probably over-strained him needlessly with my questions. After his death, which doesn't make any further impression on me, thoughts about whether the widow will stay in the palace, whether I should report his death to headquarters and, as next in command, take over the direction of the palace? Then I am standing at the window, scrutinizing the ships as they pass; they are merchant ships, roaring past rapidly on the dark waters, some of them with several funnels, others with bulging decks. . . . Then my brother is standing next to me and we are both looking out of the window onto the canal. One ship makes us start in

> alarm and call: The warship is coming. But it turns out that only the same ships already familiar to me are returning. Now there is a small ship passing by, oddly truncated, so that it ends at its broadest point; on deck there are some curious things to be seen, rather like cups and cans. We call as with one voice: *That is the breakfast-ship.*[12]

This dream, I will argue, which turns on the cost of assuming the Symbolic function in his family, differs in a number of respects from the previous dream, including the fact that the dream is so much more bellicose and in that a death appears right in the midst of it, and, as a result, we do not have to fish it out of the latent dream material. Also, we will miss quite a lot of the dream's latent meaning if we are fooled by the dream's rather heavy-handed allusion to oedipal triangles and do not inquire into what these triangles represent in the dream, and what they are trying to keep from entering consciousness.

In particular, I will argue that uncovering the death wishes in the dream will involve deciphering who the Herr P, who Freud kills with his overtaxing questions, is. That is, it requires knowing who or what the dreamer makes go away. By and by, following this line of inquiry will help us recognize how this death wish is also connected to Freud's desire to assume the Symbolic function in his family, just as it will also highlight the cost Freud pays for assuming the Symbolic function at home.

Who Herr P is, however, will be our first concern. Let us get past the obvious. The association of Herr P to Freud's father is apparent, but who else may Herr P be? Is Herr P Breuer, who rejects Freud's claim to the Symbolic function when he repudiates Freud's theories, and, hence, who is someone Freud unconsciously associates with the frustration and castration of an erotic desire? Is Herr P Fliess, who is having an operation when Freud has the dream? Is Herr P Freud's deceased friend Paneth, who Freud designates by the initial "P" in *The Interpretation of Dreams* (the "Non Vixit" dream)? Is Herr P the long dead Julius? Freud even writes that *he* may be Herr P. And, we have to admit that any and all of these men can claim a stake in Freud's unconscious wishes to assume the Symbolic function in his family, hence they all can have a role in forming the figure of Herr P in the dream. We may begin to wonder, then, to what extent Herr P is a condensation of all these figures; including a figure I have not yet mentioned—the figure of Herr P also alludes to an unconscious, that is repressed, wish to kill Eli Bernays.

Who, then, is Eli Bernays? To begin with, Eli is Freud's brother-in-law. For much of Freud's adult life, Eli also is a friend, and Eli may have introduced Freud to his younger sister, Martha Bernays, who Freud will marry following a five year engagement. But the dream also suggests that Freud harbors guilty death wishes for Eli in his unconscious too, and that these death wishes touch on Freud's conflicts over the cost of assuming the Symbolic function in his family, a price that may involve having to symbolically get rid of Eli first.

But, to explain how and why Freud harbors death wishes for Eli in his unconscious will require that we make a brief excursion into the place of the father in Freud's unconscious, and, in particular, it requires that we make inquiries into the ways that the place of the father has become linked in Freud's unconscious to "money" as an unconscious signifier of access to the Symbolic order. For, the signifier "money" binds together a whole slew of erotic wishes and death wishes connected to Freud's frustrated unconscious desire to assume the Symbolic function in the family. These worries, we know, also are rooted in real life; for, Freud faces serious, ongoing money problems throughout his childhood and student years. His poverty aggrieves him, especially, during his engagement to Martha. It also complicates his romancing of Martha, for example, when Martha's mother, hearing her daughter has gotten engaged to a penniless researcher, tries to bring Martha back to Hamburg where she can watch her daughter better. Freud, who always finds conflicts with women tricky, turns his anger against his erstwhile friend Eli instead for supporting his mother's decision to bring Martha home.

Other grievances which join together Freud's unconscious erotic frustrations and the words "money" and "Eli" follow. For example, at one point, Eli and Freud plan to have a double wedding so that Eli can marry Anna, Freud's younger sister, at the same time that Freud marries Martha, Eli's younger sister. But because of Freud's ongoing money problems, Eli goes ahead and marries Anna alone, drawing attention to Freud's impecunious finances. If this does not rankle Freud enough, Eli quickly becomes a successful businessman who can support the Bernays family after the death of Eli's father at a time when Freud's poverty means that he has to play second fiddle to Eli in family matters. His simmering hostility toward Eli breaks out when Martha gives Eli control of her inheritance to invest, and without consulting her, Freud calls Eli a scoundrel in a letter and demands he return Martha's money to her. Although Martha makes Freud apologize, he angrily accuses Eli a few years later of hiring Alexander, Freud's younger brother, and then cheating and insulting him.[13]

These are all what one may call typical family squabbles, and by the time of Freud's "breakfast ship" dream, they are a thing of the past. Freud has patched up his relationship with Eli.[14] But, by that time, Eli has already become ensconced in Freud's unconscious as a name associated with libidinal frustration. That is, the word "Eli" has become linked by that time to feelings of frustration regarding Freud's wish to assume the Symbolic function in his family and in his work life. And, furthermore, the word "Eli" has already taken its place in Freud's unconscious alongside other narcissistic grievances, experiences of castration, and the absence of Symbolic power. Remember, for example, that Freud feels he is being unfairly held at the university rank of professor *extraordinarius* at about the same time, a position that is little better than the rank of adjunct professor today, do to systemic anti-Semitism and the aristocratic-Catholic monopoly on civic and state power in the Austro-Hungarian Empire.

Thus, we can surmise that Freud feels crimped and neglected at the time he has this dream and that events in that year will remind Freud, at least unconsciously, of his earlier conflicts with Eli, who, in the meantime, has migrated to America, when Freud reads of the sinking of the Spanish fleet at San Juan, Puerto Rico, by American naval forces.[15] The outbreak of war between Spain and America, then, stirs Freud's unconscious complaints against Eli. And the result is the dream, with Eli transformed into the hapless Herr P, a figure Freud slanders as ineffectual, and who Freud's character kills off before he assumes the position of the senior officer in charge of the defense (read: as the head of the household and as the chief object of Martha's affections).

The dream, therefore, presents Eli's death as the fulfillment of a wish. In this respect, the death wish conforms in every respect to Freud's early theory of what a death wish is; and, accordingly, following Herr P's death in the dream, the ships quite literally come in, conveying a sustained image of happiness that, in the association phase of the dream, makes Freud say that he recalls a *pleasant vacation with his wife* when they witness an English warship decked in festive colors, and Martha exclaims, just as Freud and his brother do in the dream, "The warship is coming!"

Thus, a bellicose start (War is declared! Herr P collapses dead! The future looks grave and uncertain!) gives way to a happy ending in the dream so that the latent thoughts behind the dream include something like the following: "Eli, after all, has not succeeded in frustrating my happiness. Look at how nicely the ships have come in after all," a theme that Freud highlights, also, when he remembers that the appearance of the breakfast ship at the end of the dream recalls *a pleasant meal he enjoyed with his wife and children* aboard a small vessel on a canal ride in Italy.[16] But, if one accepts this reading of the dream one will be sadly disappointed to learn that, in fact, things do not end so nicely. For, Freud goes on to say, in regards to the breakfast ship and that pleasant canal ride with Martha and his children, that the breakfast ship also reminds him of a *black Etruscan breakfast table service*[17] that he sees on the same vacation during which he enjoys the breakfast ship meal with Martha and his children. And, it is at this point that the associations darken and Freud goes on to remember that the table service is "a [*schwarze Toilette*]," a *schwarze Toilette* being something that the Etruscans used while in "mourning . . . *a direct allusion to someone's death.*"[18]

To bring the point home, Freud also remembers that the word "breakfast" (as in "breakfast ship") divides into two words: breaking and fasting, with breaking recalling a breaking of a ship in the sense "of *a shipwreck*" and fasting recalling "the sense of *mourning*" to mind.[19] Read in this way, this dream is saying that the price of his happiness and of his ascension to the Symbolic function may have come at too high a price, and that a shipwreck lies at the bottom of it all.

We really are in the heart of Freudian ambivalence at this point where much of what we take for erotic satisfaction reveals itself to be founded in a repressed death wish; and, the dream suggests that assuming the position of the Symbolic father comes at a terrible cost for Freud. For, like Oedipus, he finds that once he assumes the Symbolic function that the pleasures it provides him are built over an abyss that may in the end conclude with the return of a ship of death; and Freud, or his unconscious, appears to say "look behind the happy ending, and consider the cost you have paid to assume the Symbolic function in the family. Has the cost been too great?" Certainly, these sorts of ideas will act as a reagent on Freud's original concept of what a death wish is, forcing him to stretch its meaning and rework it, for, if it is true that death wishes are desires to remove an obstacle to an erotic satisfaction, they also lead to guilt, disunion, disharmony, and death. We therefore have reached something of an impasse, where Freud's dream seems to say that one's happiness and satisfaction are floating on a sea of death.

These narratives in Freud's unconscious also emerge in the myth of the primal murder in "Totem and Taboo" (1912–1913) which portrays how the brothers, having removed their father, become a slave to their remorse and fear. Thus, although they act to set their desires free, they discover that they have not set their desires free at all, but that they instead have had to flee their own remorse and fear into an even more severe Symbolic order. Once again, we can see the question hovering behind the story: is it worth the price the subject has to pay—the installation of castration anxiety—has entering into the Symbolic order paid off? We are forced to ask this question, Freud's dream suggests because, if we look behind the wish that things have come out alright (that, indeed, the ships have come in!), we find that the dream is inferring that you cannot always get what you want, and, in this case, that the removal of an obstruction has been replaced by castration anxiety, which, in the big picture, is certainly not an improvement but may in fact be worse.

In implying all of this in the myth of the primal murder, then, Freud has greatly complicated his original view that a death wish is the wish to get rid of an obstruction to an erotic wish; it still is that, of course, but Freud's emphasis is now focused on the costs people pay to assume the Symbolic function more than it focuses on the pleasures that they accrue by fulfilling the death wish—costs which include the installation of a Symbolic order that is ground more in guilt and remorse than love, a Symbolic order to which the individual brings his or her private desires to be judged and scrutinized.

All this, writes Freud, is the legacy of the satisfaction of death wishes at some time in the past, a legacy that, Freud will add in 1923, has been taken into the psyche and turned against the ego by the superego. Of course, once people have crossed over into the Symbolic order, they cannot go back, they must go forward, and try to moderate the castration anxiety and make the Symbolic function in a less critical way. But, Freud will suggest even in 1912–1913 that the totem, as an object in the external world on which the community projects its collective father complex, stands for what is prohibited and cannot be eaten; what is sacred. But, the prohibition against eating, however, is a secondary prohibition. The first prohibition is, for Freud, a prohibition against murder because, you will recall that Freud says that the brothers kill and eat their father. The dietary prohibition, then, is a form of symbolic remembrance, that is to say, it is a symbolic remembrance and it is a prohibition against remembering the murder and the wish to murder the father at the same time; and, for this act of forgetting to be viable, the totem must also prohibit incest, since it is the incestuous wish that drives the brothers to kill their father in the first place, according to Freud.[20]

As well as becoming a dietary prohibition, the prohibition against killing also becomes associated with prohibitions against impurity and touch, since murder is, above all, an act of touching (like sex). Thus, Freud notes, under most circumstances, the totem cannot be touched and its manna kills if the clan does not obey precise prohibitions concerning its handling, or even concerning looking directly at things that share some of its power, including menstruating women and men who have killed someone. Also, to the extent that the chief partakes of the sacred power of the totem father-complex, he, too, can be approached only with caution and he becomes the aim of a great many inhibitions and restrictions that restrict and unconsciously punish him.

Each one of these taboos, however, can be violated either by special individuals or at special times in the calendar, thus revealing the nature of the Symbolic order rests on its ability to use guilt and remorse (reinforced by force) to regulate desires and to prohibit the individual and the collective from either discovering their own desire that is not given to them in the Symbolic order and to prohibit them from remembering things past except when those memories are obscured by the cloak of the Symbolic order. But, if the foundation of the Symbolic lies in taking hold of, and regulating, the sense of remorse and guilt associated with the death wish, the obvious question is why people ever give in to their death wishes in the first place and why do they put up with the restrictions and control of their death wishes and their feelings of loss? In one sense, this was the question that Wilhelm Reich came to, although from a very different starting point that includes his rejection of the idea of a death drive. For Reich believed that to become sexually healthy, people have to overthrow the restraints of the Symbolic order that have come to reside in their bodies and mind, and so realize their full libidinal potency. But, things are never that simple for Freud, for whom the answer to the question of why people do not just slough off the Symbolic ties that bind them together lies partly in the importance erotic unions have in people's lives. People, having grown up in families, want to feel united in communities that go beyond their own egos, even when the Symbolic ties produce discontent in them. But, a deeper answer lies in the suggestion that people feel that the Symbolic protects them from their own death wishes and from the consequences of their remorse.

Thus, when Freud researches into the narcissistic disorders and writes "Mourning and Melancholia" (1917), the issue behind the book is not just a desire on Freud's part to explain what is happening to object libido when libido flows to the ego (which is the question most of Freud's commentators have pursued) but a desire on Freud's part to explain why people persist in mourning a lost object when ongoing mourning turns into depression. That is, why do they, unconsciously at least, choose discontentment and sickness over letting go of the object? And, we can say now that at least part of the answer to this question for Freud is the following: that a melancholic runs the risk of arousing remorse of another loss buried in their unconscious when they let go of their remorse for the object they are consciously mourning. It is this other lost object, as much as the consciously lost one, which the melancholic does not want to think about. Because if they did, the thought would arouse a taboo and it also would generate intolerable guilt and remorse.

In this sense, melancholia performs the same defensive function as the Symbolic. In both cases, the aim is to maintain the subject in a state of constant pathological mourning. For healthy mourning, writes Freud, frees the libido that has formerly been frozen by grief so that the ego can find new objects to love, whereas the father complex has exactly the opposite effect: it draws the destructive energies unleashed in the grieving process into the regulation of the individual and the community, and, after 1923 Freud will add, punish the ego for violating real and imaginary prohibitions.

Many of these themes appear again in Freud's essay "Timely Reflections on War and Death" (1915). The aim of this essay is to answer the question of how the war has changed—or may change—the way people think about death, especially how the war may change the attitudes toward death of those civilians who are sheltered from the most direct and brutal forms of the war, people, that is, like Freud himself. Let us see what Freud writes. This large-scale exercise in blood-letting he reminds himself is being carried out and condoned by almost all of those who assume the Symbolic role in all of the nations of Europe. In this war, it is the representatives of the State, the governments of the most "civilized" nations of Europe, which legitimate and direct the most brutal acts of murder. But the individual has faired no better than the governments in this war, as even those individuals who professed the highest levels of civilization before the war are now calling for the bloody liquidation of the enemy's forces. It is, Freud suggests, a sad state of affairs all things considered were it not that the war teaches us that it was wrong to expect that most people and governments were ever very moral to begin with. Instead, the war has revealed the truth that most people do right only when they are not threatened or when they are not given permission by the Symbolic order to give vent to their death wishes. These death wishes are never gone, they are always not far below the surface, and now that the war has allowed people the release of these pent up desires at last, it has revealed how thin the cover of civilization really is for most people for whom "there is no eradication of evil. Rather . . . man's deepest essence lies in drive-impulses that are elemental in nature and identical in all people, and are aimed at the satisfaction of certain primal needs."[21] As a result," Freud writes, "a person subject to their influence decides upon good actions in the cultural sense without any ennoblement of his drives, without any transformation of egotistic into social inclinations."[22]

There moral development remains incomplete, Freud writes, and is based more on fears of being seen and punished than on a real inner need to act ethically. Society makes people pretend to be good; but, in fact, "every hour of every day, in our unconscious impulses, we remove everyone who gets in our way."[23] One should not despair at how far some people and governments have fallen then because in reality they have not fallen that far from what they were before as we imagined; they never were able to control their death wishes, and, these same people and governments who now are the loudest most bellicose voices will after the war possibly return to the level of morality that they have fallen from and perhaps may even advance from that position, having gained a new perspective in the war, to make more advances on the road to a Symbolic order rooted in tolerance. War may then establish the conditions of an inner reformation in some people's unconscious attitudes toward death and killing.

I am sure the reader has seen that this is not an appeal to war as a metaphor of psychic renewal à la Ernst Junger.[24] Freud is not speaking of the camaraderie-in-arms of soldier, of how the war strips life of all its artificiality and thrusts the individual back into an immediate, visceral life "beyond good and evil"; rather, Freud is interested in looking at how the war may weaken the repetitions of the past and clear a space for a new psychic relation to our death wishes, one where the father complex does not regulate the Symbolic forms of the death wish in the same old ways as before the war. And, apropos this, Freud will write in later texts like *Beyond the Pleasure Principle* (1920) that trauma such as the one people experienced in the last war tends to cause a regression to a primitive emotional state "beyond the pleasure principle" where efforts to contain suffering are limited to a compulsion to repeat the same painful impulse again in an attempt to prepare the ego to bring the repetition of trauma to an end the second or third time around; and so, in the fashion that he already argued for in "Mourning and Melancholia" (1917), free libido to find a new object that will permit life for the wounded ego to start again.

Freud returns to many of the same problems again, but this time from the perspective of two gifted individuals whose cultured and eroticized death wishes leave them unable to enjoy beauty, but, instead, turn them into melancholic aesthetics. Or, to say this differently, they feel the loss of the object so deeply that they experience painful signs of loss everywhere, especially in the things that, being beautiful, could arouse their libido. Thus, for these companions of Freud, death has become the object of excessive feelings of loss that has turned mourning into melancholia, but while they can see the loss inherent in all things, they cannot feel the death wish that precedes the loss, that is, their affects are deficient to the extent that they grieve but forget what they are grieving, but that, after all, is the role of the Symbolic order.

Thus, in "On Transience" (1916), Freud describes walking in the countryside of the Dolomite mountains "in the summer before the war" with: "a silent friend and a young and already well-known poet[25] . . . disturbed by the idea that all this beauty was bound to fade, that it would vanish through the winter, like all human beauty and everything beautiful and noble that people have created and would create."[26]

These gifted companions of Freud force all their desires through the millstone of grief and unresolved loss and do not mourn, for "mourning . . . comes to an end. . . . Then our libido becomes free once again."[27] Something is blocking the flow of their libido so their "revolt against grief" devalues "the pleasure of beautiful things for them"[28]—and we now can guess what that inhibition is: it is the Symbolic order itself which controls how they are grieving so that they do not remember their death wish but only recall a feeling of loss. They grieve but do not allow the death wish behind the feelings of loss to appear in consciousness. And, this is the point, this is why they can not escape from suffering. And, this also is why Freud will ask his readers: "Would it not be better," Freud concludes, "to give death the place in reality and in our thoughts that is its due, and bring out the unconscious attitudes to death, which we have hitherto so carefully suppressed, a little more?"[29]

To conclude, the reader can see, I am sure, that Freud's description of the forms that death wishes take is beginning to overwhelm the confines of his theory that death wishes are simply wishes to remove an obstacle to the satisfaction of an erotic wish, for what is there in such a theory that can help to explain the way erotic wishes are undermined by guilt and remorse, and, also, what is there in such a theory to explain the appearance in people of repressed anxieties of dying? Castration anxiety covers some of these problems, but not all of them, and, as a result, Freud's theory of what the death wish is will enter a period of flux that will be resolved by Freud only after he formulates his second metapsychology of the drives in 1920.

Another way to frame this problem is to ask why did the brothers give in to their death wish, and why do people continue to give in to them, given their negative impact on their lives? Freud really has no answer for these questions until he concludes that things have happened this way, and they continue to happen this way, because our death wishes are not only expressions of a wish to remove an obstacle to an erotic wish, but that they are also, and primarily, an expression of a drive for things to fall apart, to come undone, to unravel, and to die; an expression, that is, of a drive to disillusionment acting in combination with a countervailing impulse for union, harmony, integration, and expansion.[30] There are other limitations with Freud's first theory of what a death wish is that he will take up in his new drive theory. Namely, he will try to address the problem that the original theory is primarily an object-libido theory in that it explains a death wish as a wish to remove an object that is standing between the subject and the satisfaction of an erotic wish. However, the study of the narcissistic disorders has shown Freud that death wishes are also wishes to destroy narcissistic pleasures. In 1920, he will publish a book in which he picks up on these ideas.

NOTES

1. There is a bit of a tautology at work here with the word "anxiety" explaining the outcome of the conversion of sexual energy into nervous energy and the definition of sexual energy that has been converted into nervous energy being given as the definition of the word "anxiety."

2. Freud, *The Interpretation of Dreams*, trans. Joyce Crick (Oxford: Oxford University Press, 1999), 157.

3. We know that the Freud household remains defined by women's spaces and men's spaces. It is Martha's responsibility to run the kitchen and oversee the mak-

ing of the dishes. Freud does not interfere in this area of domestic life but waits till a bell rings when he leaves his office and enters the dining area where Martha and the children are waiting for him. Both Freud and Martha enjoy this middle-class way of ordering their domestic life, and we can presume that Freud experienced a similar arrangement in his parent's home. Katja Behling, *Martha Freud, A Biography*, trans. R. D. V. Glasgow (New York: Polity, 2006).

4. Deborah Margolis, *Freud and His Mother: Pre-oedipal Aspects of Freud's Personality* (Lanham, Md.: Jason Aronson Press, 1977).

5. Louis Breger, *Freud: Darkness in the Midst of Vision—An Analytic Biography* (Hoboken, N.J.: Wiley, 2000).

6. Freud, *The Interpretation of Dreams*, 195.

7. In *The Interpretation of Dreams* Freud labels these sorts of death wishes in dreams as "typical dreams." And, he seems intent on stressing how common, and in some sense inconsequential, these death wishes are in childhood.

8. Sigmund Freud, "Femininity" (1931) in *The Standard Edition* 21:223–43. Quoted in Breger, *Darkness*, 13–14.

9. On September 29, 1896, he writes Fliess: "I would like so much to hold out until the famous age limit of approximately fifty-one . . . but I had one day that made me feel it was unlikely." Jeffrey Mousaieff Masson, ed., *The Complete Letters of Sigmund Freud to Wilhelm Fliess Correspondences* (Cambridge, Mass.: Belknap Press of Harvard University Press, 1986).

10. Sigmund Freud, "Sexuality and the Aetiology of the Neuroses," in *The Standard Edition of the Complete Psychological Works of Sigmund Freud* vol. 3 (New York: W. W. Norton & Co., 1976), 189–221.

11. Fleischl's death lies in the background of a number of Freud's dreams in the later 1890s, and Fleischl appears clearly in the manifest content of the famous "Non Vixit" dream which concerns Freud's anxiety for his friend Fliess who has recently undergone a serious operation, and for a series of other men whom Freud feels affection and who have died. The dream begins: "I had gone to Brucke's laboratory at night, in response to a gentle knock on the door; I opened it to the late Professor Fleischl who came with a number of strangers and, after exchanging a few words, sat down at his table."

12. Freud, *The Interpretation of Dreams*, 301–302.

13. Behling, *Martha Freud*, 55–59.

14. Indeed, Freud will retain an aversion to poverty all his life.

15. Patricia Gherovici discusses the connection between the newspaper reports Freud reads about the Spanish and American naval battle at San Juan and this dream in Gherovici, *The Puerto Rican Syndrome* (London: The Other Press, 2003). Freud's identification with Spanish literature, and his dislike of America, may reinforce his old rivalry with Eli over money and Martha's affections.

16. In *The Puerto Rican Syndrome*, Gherovici writes that the breakfast ship may also allude to Scott's cessation of the naval battle so that breakfast could be eaten.

17. In the dream: "On the deck there are some curious things to be seen, rather like cups and cans."

18. Freud, *The Interpretation of Dreams*, 301.

19. Freud, *The Interpretation of Dreams*, 304.

20. Ambivalence and identification are the keys to the father complex, according to Freud. Thus, in Freud's construction, the clan behaves as if the totem is something loved and hated, protecting and dangerous at the same time. The clan treats the totem as an object of idealized veneration, and identification most of the time. If it is an animal, no clan person may kill or eat it. But the clan also treats the totem as if it is strange and dangerous, and, therefore, an incitement to forbidden and licentious impulses that must be held in check because they partake of the prohibited thing—the memory-traces of a murdered or vengeful father.

21. Freud, "A Timely Reflection of War and Death," in *On Murder, Mourning, and Melancholia*, trans. Michael Hulse (London: Penguin Classics, 2005), 175.

22. Freud, "A Timely Reflection on War and Death," 178.

23. Freud, "A Timely Reflection on War and Death," 190–191. Also see Sigmund Freud, *Totem and Taboo* in *The Complete Psychological Works of Sigmund Freud*, vol. 13 (New York: W. W. Norton & Co., 1976) where Freud argues that people only learn to fear their own death by experiencing the death of a loved one.

24. Someone like Nietzsche initially welcomes the wars of the 1860s and the Franco-Prussian war (1870) because he sees war casting the superior soul into the Hericlitian whirlpool of Being that exists behind the world of representations. But Nietzsche becomes horrified when the wars lead not to the rejuvenation of culture but to nationalism and militarism. Rudiger Safranski, *Nietzsche: A Philosophic Biography*, trans. Shelley Frisch (New York: W. W. Norton & Co., 2003), 85–86.

25. The two companions may be Lou Andreas Salome and Maria Rilke, although the veracity of the walk has been questioned by authors recently.

26. Freud, "On Transience" (1916) in *On Murder, Mourning, and Melancholia*, 197.

27. Freud, "On Transience,"199–200.

28. Freud, "On Transience," 198.

29. Freud writes: "Death can no longer be denied."

30. Another piece of this revision will happen when, by placing the superego over the ego and the id in his new structural theory, Freud grounds the Law, the prohibition against certain desires, in the constant scrutinizing of the ego for signs of guilt.

3

Freud's Later Views Concerning Death as a Drive

How much must these people have suffered to achieve such beauty!

—Nietzsche, *The Birth of Tragedy*

One way to think about what happens to Freud's work in 1920 is to say that he replaces libido theory with a new dual drive theory. And, while this is fundamentally correct, it is even more correct to say that Freud never really gives up on libido theory, but that he sees it operating within a larger drive theory in which organisms are pulled between urges to come undone and die and to unite and live. Another way to say this is that after 1920 the distinctive change in Freud's work is not that he rejects libido theory but that he feels compelled to tinker with and change parts of it so that he can introduce his new notion—that new notion being that a death wish is more than a representation of a wish to remove an obstruction to an erotic wish, it also is a representation of the interactions of Eros, or the urge to union and integration, with a death drive to make things fall apart and eventually die. But the meaning of this other change depends on what a death drive is. This chapter, therefore, will focus on Freud's effort to answer the question of what a death drive is, with the warning at the start of the chapter that the answer Freud gives to the question of what a death drive is remains incomplete, but that this is something that Freud knew all too well himself.

To begin with a little review, before the development of the dual drive theory in 1920, Freud's overarching explanation of the drives is contained in his libido drive theory. But what libido theory actually says is not completely clear. Drive theory, Freud says time and time again, is at once the most speculative and least worked out portions of psychoanalytic theory because it belongs to the level of an explanatory system of clinical data (Freud's metapsychology) rather than to the descriptive level of clinical data. Nevertheless, Freud professes his belief that no one can make sense of psychic life without developing an explanation for the drives, and any psychological explanation of the drives would be inadequate without a view of how the drives are related to the unconscious representations of words and images. The importance of drives and the importance of understanding their relation to language appears quite early in Freud's thinking, but they do not go back to its beginning, being held by Freud certainly no later than the mid-1890s when he writes his aphasia paper and when he fails to explain the neurological pathways underlying language use and affects. Freud maintains the sense that drives are a mysterious and heterodox substance throughout his life. They originate in the body, especially in the various erotic zones of the body, but it would be a mistake to tie them too closely to those body zones since each and every one of the drives also has a representational form, which the drive can utilize in order to displace a drive from one body zone to another body zone and from one object to another.

Freud also says that drives occupy a space intermediary to the body and the mind. Drives also seem to Freud to have a mysterious property of being able to convert their energy from sexual to asexual energy or from sexual energy to anxiety, for example. But this is not surprising given the fact that drives had a hybrid psychosexual nature for Freud from the start. Since the drives are forms of psychosexual energy, Freud wants to understand by what principles and by means of what psychological mechanisms can the energy levels of the drives rise and fall. Also, Freud wants to distinguish between the source of a drive (usually a body zone), the aim of the drive, and the object of the drive. Thus, he suggests the drives can be separated by sources and aims into two opposing groupings. The first set of drives seeks the discharge of libido originating in the body; these drives are libido drives and they seek pleasure, by discharging pent-up sexual tensions. The second set of drives aims to preserve the life of the individual. These drives also originate in the body. They are collectively called by Freud the self-preservative or ego drives and they include things like hunger, the urge to sleep, and so on.

Thus, in Freud's first drive theory, people are motivated by opposing urges of love and hunger. Libido also has a second species-wide aim, and that is the reproduction of the species, which can sometimes stand in opposition to the pleasure-seeking drives. But this is an old story, and it is no stranger to speak of libido having opposing aims than it is to speak of the fact that one form of pleasure-seeking in an organism will oppose another. Nor is it any stranger to speak of competing libidinal drives than it is to speak of the fact that one form of pleasure-seeking may reinforce the ego drives while another does just the opposite. Nevertheless, both the pleasure-seeking and the reproductive urges regularly place libido in conflict with the ego drives, and this becomes the principle demarcation line between the drives. On one side of the line for Freud are the libido drives and on the other side of the line are the ego drives.

Thus, although the number of separate drives, in fact, is potentially limitless, Freud organizes them around the aims of sexual discharge (pleasure) and self-preservation; he organizes them, that is, around the antimony of love and hunger. Then, in 1920, the way Freud explains the drives and their relation to (and place in) the psychic apparatus changes. Now, the potentially limitless number of drives is organized (unified) around the aims of two new impulses. The first drive aims to sustain life by uniting substances into greater and greater wholes. While this drive, the life drive, is closely allied with the pleasure principle, it also can oppose it, when, for example, the love between two people stands in the way of a person's cultural work. Nevertheless, the telos of Eros is to seek larger and more inclusive groups that bind the individual to networks. The other drive is a drive to disintegrate ties between people and things and to speed up the slide back to death and the return to the inorganic world by decomposing or breaking up the unions that sustain and increase the diversity of life. Hence, when it can, the death drive seeks the breakdown of groups, it works to make things fall apart and come undone. Finally, both Eros and the death drive share a common aim of reducing psychic tensions, but they seek to reduce psychic tension by pursuing diametrically opposite courses of action, and both Eros and, paradoxically, the death drive are liable to be the source of heightened neuroses and suffering since there are so many competing drives, and since the satisfaction of a drive always comes up against the limits of the Symbolic order, the desires of other people, and the limitations of Nature.

Freud introduces the dual drive theory in *Beyond the Pleasure Principle* (1920) with all sorts of misgivings. The notion that the old dualism of love and hunger be replaced by one of union and disunion (or life and death) is a sort of thought experiment, he writes a bit defensively, to see how far the idea can go. Very soon, however, Freud gives up his doubts and he never wavers afterward in his adherence to the new dualist model.

The period of his greatest doubts appear to have only lasted between 1920 and 1924. By that time, Freud already has concluded that if a drive to destroy the subject exists then there also has to be a primary masochism, too. Freud, therefore, concludes that his prior belief that masochism was a secondary response to sadism has to be wrong. Or, rather, it had seemed logical before to believe that sadism is the more primary form hate assumes, if for no other reason than that, as a wish to remove an obstruction to an erotic wish, a death wish had seemed a sadistic act, and not a masochistic one, the urge only becoming masochistic when the original wish to remove the object is turned back onto the ego as in melancholia by guilt or by some other defense mechanism like splitting. All this begins to change when Freud examines the narcissistic disorders, because the aetiological picture begins to look far more complicated. But, the old theory that masochism is a response to a death wish turned against the ego only becomes indefensible once Freud switches to the dual drive theory which assumes an independent drive to destroy the subject exists but precedes the ego turning its erotic and destructive urges against an object. Consequently, Freud begins to write as if the ego has a primal masochism, although he does not deny the existence of secondary forms of masochism either that arise when sexual sadism is turned inward again. Moral masochism typifies this form of secondary masochism. It, therefore, is not the case that Freud no longer believes in masochism secondary to a sadistic wish, rather it is simply the case that he now rethinks the meaning of secondary masochism in light of a preexisting primary masochism.

At this point, someone may wonder what Freud hopes to do by modifying his views in such a radical direction. Why does he not just let well enough alone and stick with a libido theory that he has developed for twenty years; for, even with its limitations, libido theory has proven itself sturdy and useful enough to explain a wide variety of contending and contradictory psychoanalytic facts. Why does Freud bother to modify the libido theory then with a new explanation of the two drives? What exactly is Freud trying to explain by replacing the dualism of love and hunger with the dualism of union and disunion?

The question is not so easy to answer and it has puzzled many of Freud's readers for a long time. As a result, when facing the inexplicable, many have manifestly rejected the whole idea of a death drive. Some simply return to libido theory and they do not see any break between it and the new dual drive theory. Others believe the second drive theory to be a great mistake, which people would do well to avoid. Only a few analysts, including Melanie Klein, have launched their own investigation of the psychic apparatus starting from it.

Some have tried to explain why Freud is drawn to a death drive. Thus, when commentators mention that the investigation of the narcissistic disorders cause Freud to believe that libido theory requires revision by the middle 1910s, the problem with this explanation is that it explains why Freud wants to modify libido theory but it does not explain why he begins to think in terms of a death drive. Others point to the impact of World War I, the economic and political upheavals after the war, the tragic death of Freud's favorite child of influenza in 1919–1920, and Freud's age, and they conclude that all of these factors are weighing on Freud and that he is becoming fatigued and worn down by life. According to this argument, Freud's more pessimistic theory conforms to his own growing pessimism, the problem with this argument being that it does not take seriously Freud's new found interest in answering the question of what a death drive is and how a death drive may interact with a drive for unity, therefore it is an incomplete answer at best.

These commentators are right about one thing, however; if we are to take Freud's new found enthusiasm for the notion of a death drive seriously we have to start by making a few comments on his character. By all accounts, Freud was a very fastidious man. Once he wrote that a person who goes out in public unkempt does so in order to express his contempt for others. He always dressed carefully and he trimmed his beard regularly at the barber. He also is purported to have liked working on a schedule. He, for instance, worked in his study everyday seeing patients, reading, or writing until a bell announced dinner. He also took regular and vigorous walks around the Ringstrasse to keep fit, and he planned all his vacations down to the smallest detail months in advance, paying special attention to train schedules.

If one likes, these are bourgeois character traits. And, in line with this explanation, Freud is said to have taken care to guarantee the financial well-being of his wife and children in the circumstance of his sudden death. But this side of his personality stands in contrast to a more rebellious side of his character which he said made him identify with the great explorers of the past and also made him an admirer of the conquistadors. This side of his personality burnt with fury when he confronted a group of anti-Semites as a student at The University of Vienna, and it also made him identify with Semitic heroes from the Bible like Moses and from the ancient world like Hannibal.

Experience teaches Freud, too, that things in this world are constantly falling apart or being threatened by disillusion, that the work of civilization is constantly unraveling, that people live lives that frequently feel as if they are coming undone. If this seems to be an excessively pessimistic account, consider the fact that between 1914 and 1920 Freud sees the devastation of the war, the capture of one of his sons on the Italian front near the end of the war, the disruption of mail service and the everyday conveniences during the war and in the chaotic years following the ending of hostilities, the near death of Martha and the loss of his favorite child in the influenza epidemic of 1919–1920, the loss of his personal savings in the economic collapse at the end of the war, the fall of the Hohenzollern, Romanov, and Hapsburg dynasties, and so on.

Other disruptions can be mentioned but it would not add to the main point which is simply that what the times call for, and what Freud feels compelled to provide the times, is an analytically sophisticated explanation of a worldwide experience of things coming undone. Libido theory is simply not an adequate theory to answer this question, whereas the dual drive theory is at least able to explain these phenomena as the byproduct of opposing urges to union and disintegration.

In other words, the wisdom of the dual drives is comparable to the wisdom that says that life is inescapably bound up in mourning; and that each and every act of Eros that binds us together also binds us to loss and to the inevitable Fate of things falling apart—and not just because all things are mortal and so will fade away in time but they also will inevitably unravel because we ourselves are pushed and pulled by urges to ruin and destroy what we build, to rush the process of disintegration that will happen in any case. We, in other words, are not merely passive victims of death but are actively engaged in it alongside our struggles to limit it and to expand the dominion of life. Given this, the question for Freud is how people relate to the losses they face and that they summon from within themselves; this is the work of masochism I spoke about earlier.

At this juncture it may be helpful to recall what I said in the previous chapter on the subject of what a death wish is. You will recall that I said there that Freud begins his work with the simple definition that a death wish is a wish to remove an obstruction to the satisfaction of an erotic wish. But very quickly, he begins to complicate this picture and eventually he arrives at the idea that the formation of the Symbolic function is based on turning the remorse and the guilt unleashed by the death wish and the deed back against the subject so that a prohibition will emerge that can guarantee the continuing repression of the remembrance of the death wish and the incestuous wish. Now, in 1920, Freud begins to tell his readers that their lives are governed not only by a regime of guilt built on top of a death wish but he also tells them that their lives are governed by the intermingling of urges to unite with others and by impulses to rush toward destruction, decay, and death. That is, Freud tells them that death affects their lives because it is a forbidden wish associated with a repressed memory-trace. But he also tells them that death affects them because it is a drive. And, if we bring these two theories together, one a theory of what a death wish is and the other a theory of what a death drive is, then Freud appears to be saying this: that basing our psychic development and building our civilization on a denial—a denial that we have ever wished to get rid of the father (the death wish)—leads not only to a higher rate of neuroses in all kinds of individuals but it also leads to having to disavow a large part of who we are, of what constitutes us as desiring subjects, and of what makes up our unconscious lives.

Thus, by advancing the dual drive theory, Freud provides a new answer to the question of what distinguishes unconsciousness and the consciousness to the degree that humans have developed a hyper-consciousness to maintain the wish to kill the father and to sleep with their mother under the bar of repression—consciousness, then, has evolved, much like the Symbolic order, to keep the memory of the wish and the deed out of our thoughts. The dual drive theory also offers an explanation of how the unconscious can be organized around the remembrance and the repetition of a loss, that is, how the unconscious becomes structured around an act of mourning.

Saying that the dual drive theory suggests that the unconscious is structured around the remembrance and repetition of an act of mourning may sound too anthropomorphic; and if we want to understand what a death drive is in Freud's mind, we have to do as he does and link psychology to biology and to evolutionary theory, and, in fact, to search for an explanation that makes sense both psychologically and biologically for why an organism would evolve a structure that repeats an inner conflict between urges toward union and disunion in the first place that would in time evolve into a conflict riddled by remorse and guilt in a semi-conscious creature. Evolutionarily speaking, then, we need to pursue a path taken by Freud and try to figure out why life would evolve a death drive. Or, to say this in a different way, evolutionarily speaking again, how and why would humans develop a civilization and a sense of morality over the last thousands of years based on the guilt and remorse associated with loss?

One of the first problems Freud sets for himself, then, when he tries to explain what a death drive is, involves explaining how a drive toward destruction and disunion is conceivable at all given what we know about evolution as a process of natural selection and the survival of the fittest. At this juncture, it may be helpful to recall that Freud already has written quite a lot on the question of the relation between the biological base of the drives in the body and the psychological base of the drives in word-representations and image-representations so that this sort of problem had occupied him in some form or other virtually from the start in the 1890s as a problem of the first rank.

Much of this work, of course, necessarily remains speculative. But this does not deter Freud from beginning at the beginning. In the distant past, Freud writes, a spark of life mysteriously appears in the dead inorganic world that has existed since the dawn of the universe. Some stimulation or change in the environment must have caused this qualitative transformation, but we know nothing about it. Nevertheless, without this stimulation, there would have been no impetus for inorganic matter to alter itself in such a way as to acquire the quality of life.

The earliest cells, suggests Freud, are born and die in an instant, since they emerge in a fundamentally hostile environment and they possess no defenses against toxins, just as the American Indians who died in droves possessed no defenses against the germs brought to America by the first Europeans, and: "For a long time, perhaps, living substance is thus being constantly created afresh and easily dying."[1] The sources of the creative and destructive processes cannot simply have been external to the organism, however. Once life emerges, there also are toxins building up within the organisms; biochemical process and morphological systems that in the organism wear down over time and stop its functioning. Thus, life can be cut short prematurely by excessive external stimuli, or it can die a natural death when the parts that make up the organism wear down of their own accord and can no longer be rejuvenated by sexual intermingling of substances or by some other action, or the organism can die prematurely due to internal processes of pathogenesis. But the real point Freud wants to make in this discussion, I think, is that there are, therefore, urges inherent in life to return to the inorganic world, to stop the biochemical processes and structures supporting life. Moreover, writes Freud, these processes of decay, of breakdown, and of corruption are not just the result of fatigue of the living substance, but this also represents an inherent impulse in life to return to a prior state of its existence and, ultimately, an urge in all life to return to an inorganic world where it will not feel pain or loss, where it cannot be disturbed by stimuli or by absence of any kind.[2] Hence in cell life: "The libido meets the instinct of death, or destruction, which is dominant in them and which seeks to disintegrate the cellular organism and to conduct each separate unicellular organism (composing it) into a state of inorganic stability (relative though this may be)."[3] Freud goes on to say: "The emergence of life will thus be the cause of the continuation of life and also at the same time of the striving toward death; and life itself will be a conflict and compromise between these two trends"[4] because Nature can know nothing of a death drive until the first inorganic compounds acquire the quality of life.[5]

At this point, the reader may want to pause and say to himself that this is a very nice story, but what is the point? The point of creating this theory, I want to suggest, is that it allows Freud to create a structure that can support a viable explanation of the appearance of a death drive at the inception of life. For, on the face of things, there is no inherent reason why life, once it is called into existence, should require an opposite drive to return life to the inorganic world—why, that is, life should not evolve mechanisms that allow it to be immortal. But, where has anyone seen immortal life? It seems on the face of things far more reasonable to believe in the existence of processes which aim to push life back into the mute world of the inorganic, that life as a biological process is intertwined with death as its opposite number and its shadow. Such a position then would have the added bonus of supporting the findings of psychoanalysis, too, which shows how the wish to be immortal is an illusion.

Thus, both biologically and psychologically speaking, Freud suggests, people are more justified to believe that death lies at the heart of life—not just as a wish but also as a drive—than to believe in an immortal soul, so that the real problem we have to ask ourselves is not how can we not believe in the immortality of the soul but why can anyone believe in it? Who has ever seen a life that is not joined to death? And, given this, one can say that Freud's idea that civilization, morality, and, indeed, all of life, is found in the repression of a death wish and incestuous desires appears less strange than the claim that humans are immortal, which is something no one has ever seen; similarly, Freud's assertion that all drives seek to return to early stages in their development, and that all drives strive to return eventually to an inorganic state, seems to be the height of common sense compared to the belief that the living can become ghosts and spirits.

The actual problem is not how Freud can think the way he does, but how reasonable people can go on denying the essence of his position, unless they have some powerful internal resistance that is keeping them from it. And, in fact, psychoanalysis supports the belief that were people to make a realistic assessment of what a death wish is and what a death drive is many would find it an absurd idea and prefer to hold onto their illusions. For, life in this Freudian world is inherently contradictory, with the urge to die being an open scandal and contradiction to the urge to life in us; the death wish, then, is a scandal not just because many people carry in their unconscious memories of forbidden death wishes and erotic wishes; there is ambivalence built right into the heart of life, and people only make themselves sicker when they try to distort or deny this fact to themselves; yet, this is just what people do—they build worlds to forget their forbidden erotic and death wishes.[6]

On a historical note, this interest in expressing natural selection in the language of nature philosophy bears comparison to a number of other first-generation psychoanalysts like Jung, Stekel, Reik, and Andreas-Salome. Thus, both Jung and Stekel embrace comparable ideas. However, their overall systems look very different, with Stekel arguing that the anxiety neuroses are representations of life and death forces in 1906.[7] Theodore Reik, a more literary man then Stekel, echoes his wish to unify the works of Freud and Nietzsche when he argues, in the October 1911 meeting of the Wednesday society, that sex and death are deeply intermingled forces in the psyche. Alfred Adler too, while not stressing the fusion of death and sexuality, argues so adamantly that Freud should accept his idea that people have an aggressive will to power that seeks to compensate for organ defects like bad eyes or being short that Eduard Hitschman complains he is a one-pony act. Ernst Jones, Sandor Ferenczi, Otto Grosz, Lou-Andreas Salome, and Sabina Spielrien also write or speak about the fusion of representations of sexuality and death at about the same time but without challenging the primacy of libido theory as directly as do Stekel, Adler, Rank, and Jung.

All this raises the question of the relation between the death wish, the death drive, and desire, too. To raise the question of desire, however, is ultimately to raise the question of language and the unconscious, for, as Lacan sees, language represents, and representation is a form of substitution, a placing of a symbol in place of something else that is not there. The structure of language, too, is diacritical so that the meaning we ascribe to a word, let us say the word "bird," is a set containing the things that everything else that is "not bird" is excluded. "Bird" has a meaning then only because we can compare it to the whole class of other "not bird" meanings. Also, words like "bird" have a metonymic meaning as well that allows them to be associated to other words that we connect to it like "flying," for example. Language, in other words, is a system of symbolic meanings that depends on lack and substitution, or absence, of something; and, as such, it is ideal for representing the loss and remorse caused by the death wish and it is equally ideal for representing the need to repress signs of the death drive by substituting a symbol for it.

Language is, however, distinct from desire. For, to desire is to long for what is not there. What in language is occluded by the sign is the longing by the subject for what it lacks and does not have; that is, what it lacks in the sense of what it cannot have because it is forbidden. Apropos this, as children, we cannot structure our own lives and so we have to let our parents structure it for us; we therefore learn to desire what it is we think they desire for us whether that is good or ill. But part of becoming an adult involves expanding desire to include not just what the other wants us to do but in deciding what it is we desire and then going out and realizing that wish to the best of our ability given the circumstances of our lives; and, for an adult to submit to the desire of someone else all of the time is an emasculating experience. We now can see that, for Freud, the thing that comes between us and our desire often is our death wishes and our death drive, especially our death drive, which constantly causes our plans to unravel and end badly. This is one reason that we require illusions, especially illusions that we, or someone, can conquer death, or at least that someone can conquer the guilt and remorse about death.

But, if belief in an after-life is an illusion, so that people can accept it as a fact only by replacing what they can truly see is there by an illusion, where can the individual see the operation of the life and death drive in the internal struggles of, for example, a modern individual? Freud offers one example of a person struggling with remorse and guilt for a repressed death wish, as well as struggling with a desire of the approval of the Other, the Symbolic order, and a wish to find his own path to his desire, in his essay on masochism (1924) and also in his depiction of the Russian writer Dostoevsky (1925) as a genius who suffers from guilt and remorse in a particularly striking way. For Dostoevsky is one of those people, writes Freud, who has an excessively strong eroticized death wish that he can keep under repression only by falling sick with a variety of symptoms. These symptoms arise out of the clash between Dostoevsky's death wish and his saintly impulses. This opposition produces so much tension in his psyche that, as an adult, he develops a gambling mania and a willingness to submit himself to the Church and State. But, even earlier, this state of internal conflict leads him to develop hallucinatory and hysterical symptoms including epilepsy and persecutory anxiety, which, in turn, causes him to fear the reprisal of his father, death wishes that were turned against himself in the image of a father thundering: "You wanted to kill your father in order to be your father yourself. Now you are your father, but a dead father. . . . Now your father is killing you."[8]

That is, Dostoevsky is overcome by guilt and remorse and by the wish to free himself from the guilt of the symbolic order so he can realize his own desire, and, as a result, the great writer develops a fear that he will die in his sleep as a child. Freud admits his helplessness when it comes to explaining how someone like Dostoevsky can turn his own inner demons into literature, proving that the rise in psychic tension, and the longing to reduce it, need not have the outcome of producing a symptom; art, in other words, saves Dostoevsky from being just a great moral masochist. The best we can do, he writes, is to provide the rather inadequate explanation about how Dostoevsky by dint of his personality and gifts manages to relieve himself from time to time of his guilt and remorse by the power of his imagination. In other words, Dostoevsky succeeds in seizing hold of his own impulses to smash up, break down, and crash and utilizing them for work only by creating an imaginary world. He is, therefore, able to find an arena to play with the same erotic wishes, death wishes, and impulses toward union and self-destruction that normally lead him to act self-destructively. But his relief is only temporary, and periods of writing remain balanced against the return of symptoms in his gambling mania, epilepsy, and so on.

What Dostoevsky's genius suggests is that people find themselves placed under such terrible internal strain, that they are oppressed by an inner feeling of danger which they desperately struggle to escape from, a feeling of being hounded by the Other and of things constantly breaking apart. Apropos this, Freud stresses in his second anxiety theory[9] that anxiety does not just arise from the conversion of inhibited libido into anxiety. It also, and perhaps primarily, signifies the presence of something *dangerous to the ego* which mobilizes the ego defenses of fight or flight and which is accompanied by a rise in psychic tension and unpleasure. And, in his discussion of this internal anxiety source, Freud stresses its similarity to and difference from the fear an animal has when in the presence of a feared object like a lion. The presence of the lion triggers fight or flight mechanisms, whose primary purpose is to remove the subject from the proximity of the source of danger. But, with anxiety, Freud writes, there is often no such object. Freud's point is that anxiety responds to internal rather than external objects, but in his studies on masochism and mourning he already had made the different but related point that the place of the object may also be left empty—that is the object generating anxiety my be a lost object.[10] And, since the source of the anxiety is often an objectless, inner fear, the ego cannot get free of the source of anxiety except by repressing it, by sublimating it, or (this is the subject of the book) by generating symptoms or inhibitions.

The reader, however, I am sure, has already deduced that this inner anxiety describes the state of mind of someone who is trapped in perpetual mourning; and, apropos this, Freud goes on to say in *Inhibition, Symptom, Anxiety* (1925) that the sources of anxiety are many, but that due to the way these fears have developed in humans they tend to become unified over time into an unconscious fear of castration—that is, of lacking something.[11]

Thus, castration gives a human form to the generalized fear of anxiety by signifying what lies behind the anxiety—the empty space where the father was but where now there is only a symbol, a prohibition, and the traces of guilt and remorse; Freud's theory of castration as a form of anxiety, in other words, establishes a trans-generational narrative explaining how the unconscious is structured around the need to mourn in perpetuity the loss of the object out of a sense of guilt and remorse.

In other words, anxiety is originally a fear that cannot be overcome by simply fighting or fleeing the feared thing because the feared thing is a repressed memory of a death wish and an act. Already, in *Mass Psychology* (1921), written in the wake of widespread right-wing backlashes against the Communist and Socialist successes of 1919–1920, as mobs of veterans standing for right-wing and left-wing revolutions battle in the streets of eastern and central Europe, Freud describes how certain organizations of masses (Eros), that are structured hierarchically like the Church and Army, turn their inner erotic urges to unite with each other toward a common ego ideal and turn their other urges to destroy and disable these unions against common external enemies; how, that is, an erotic bond is forged and maintained between the masses by directing their longing for a father onto a common ego ideal and their longing to smash and destroy the unions that sustain life against a stranger.

This human—all too human—desire to project the impulse to destroy and to disunite onto an external enemy constitutes an effort by Eros and the death drive to carve out spaces of their own. For, what else is this urge to be rid of the impulse to destroy and disunite, by externalizing it against a stranger, than a displacement of the urge to be free of castration anxiety in one's relation to the other members of the community onto a different scene? It amounts to a failed adjustment to create a space of safety free of the urge to destroy where people's narcissistic libidos can be given full rein vis-à-vis a common leader or ideal. The real thing binding the community together then for Freud is the ability of the group to collectively cover their death wish for the father by turning the remorse, guilt, and anger they feel against the stranger. The common ego ideal is at once a form of unacknowledged mourning and a means of taking the emotions aroused in the act of mourning and turning them against those who remain outsiders.

Freud then seems to say that these unions have to be paid for by turning the destructive impulses outside and that the function of the ideal is to bind all the members to one another by giving them a common point of identification for love and for hate. Such unions, however, remain fragile in their own ways, depending on the scene of mourning being kept under repression, as well as depending on having an other to hate. Otherwise, the death drive may overwhelm the erotic bonds linking the members to one another, and to a common ego ideal, and this usually results in a rise in aggression being directed inward again.

We do not wish to look at our existence like this, however, because it offends our narcissism, and it fills our minds with horror. And, in reality, civilization blunders forward and, in *The Future of an Illusion* (1928), Freud expresses the hope that scientific culture can sublimate (desexualize) the destructive impulses in ways that are suited to a tolerant world committed to the discovery of the truth more than religious culture was, science being a vast and glorious experiment in submitting desire to the discipline of the reality principle for Freud.

Hence, Freud suggests that we do make progress, despite our need to fall and be disunited, we manage to form unions, sublimate mourning into beauty, and so on. But this optimism already fades when Freud writes *Civilization and Its Discontents* (1930)—Freud's most pessimistic book—published in the same year as the first Nazi electoral successes that will sweep Hitler's party into political power in the 1932 German national elections. "Men are not gentle creatures," writes Freud there, "who want to be loved, and who at most can defend themselves if they are attacked; they are, on the contrary, creatures among whose intellectual endowments is to be reckoned a powerful share of aggressiveness. . . . *Homo homini lupus*."[12] For, the urge to unite is always opposed by a counter-urge to exploit and destroy the other; and, while the structure in which Eros is completed by a death drive is a natural one, Freud suspects that it has become a pathological compulsion to repeat an unfinished act of mourning.

Freud describes an individual as a being caught between the pressure to desexualize his impulses and by his ongoing attachments to sexual and narcissistic aims. We already have seen this position when he complains in "On War" that most people only act morally out of a fear of punishment while secretly continuing to crave the satisfaction of all their erotic and destructive wishes; that, in fact, the Symbolic only takes hold of the desire of the individual to make the individual desire what the Symbolic wants him to desire through a combination of fear, guilt, and remorse. And Freud's explanation of how and why such a system functions is that the individual and the collective need to mourn perpetually and to do something with the guilt and remorse that mourning elicits in them.

Thus, in the mid-1920s, for example, Freud writes an article on character types who, in some fashion, are the victims of a too punitive or a too lax ego ideal. These reflect minds that are constantly tripping up, whose sense of their own desire has been distorted into a seeming wish to gratify the Other by enacting a breakdown of some sort, that is, of characters whose Eros has become intertwined with the death drive. Thus, Freud mentions people who follow each and every success with a failure, criminals who, having gotten away, get caught, and:

> People all of whose human relationships have the same outcome: such as the benefactor who is abandoned in anger after a time by each of his protégés, however much they may differ from one another, and who thus seems doomed to taste all the bitterness of ingratitude; or the man whose friendships all end in betrayal by his friends; or the man who time after time in the course of his

life raises someone else into a position of great private or public authority and then, after a certain interval, himself upsets that authority and replaces him by a new one.[13]

In other words, to satisfy the desire of the Other for things to fall apart, they follow a success with a failure. In this regard, Freud also mentions lovers who repeatedly raise someone to a position of great personal authority and significance and then sacrifice their relationship. That is, he refers to people who find an unconscious compulsion to repeat the act of loss, but while they feel all the complex feelings of anger, betrayal, self-incrimination that we associate with mourning, they remain unaware of this fact.

By highlighting this dynamic in Freud's work, I am trying to focus on a certain relation that exists between the conscious and the unconscious states of desire. That is, that a clash between union and disunity on the drive level is being expressed at the unconscious level of desire by means of a compulsion to repeat inscribed in the unconscious as a representation of trauma but that enters consciousness only as a symptom.[14]

The notion that the unconscious, including the oedipal form of the unconscious, is repeating a pathological act of mourning helps to explain why so many people prefer comforting illusions like the illusion of an after-life. Doing so simply requires the subject rely on their pleasure principle. And, one would expect that a mind structured by the repressed need to mourn would be the sort of mind which would generate illusions of being immortal, too. Thus, as we have already seen, the oedipal complex itself is such a fantasy based on the presentation of the guilt and remorse minus the remembrance of the death wish.

All this suggests that the clashes between Eros and the death drive occurring in the unconscious take the form of a trauma and also take the form of an act of forgetting; but it also suggests that the clashes between the unconscious compulsion to mourn and the conscious production of illusions of even those who face their own death and the loss of those they love soberly must fight against the return of these unconscious fantasies of mourning and death, as even Freud saw in a letter to Arnold Zweig soon after undergoing another cancer operation on his mouth when he exclaims:

What is happening to me? I am submitting to nature, which is letting me age faster in the last three months than in the previous three years. Everything around me is gloomy, stifling to the point of choking. Fury is mounting and gnawing away at the core. If only I can do something liberating![15]

The tension bound up in the clash of the dual drive in us cannot be overcome easily. Our fear of dying may throw us into a state of terror and cause us to revert to old memory-traces and psychic forms that we thought we had given up, but which are still being cathected in the wake of the trauma situation inside us as repressed thoughts and feelings. The neurotic then is someone who remains stuck in a certain kind of exchange with their death wishes and their death drive since, for the neurotic—and this is even more so the case for the schizophrenic—death is too close, and because it is too near, it must be covered up by illusions, or symptoms.

All of this suggests that people rarely find the happiness they search for in the world satisfying for long because nature and other people conspire against it. Not only is there an inner drive to disunion, decomposition, and death, but this drive has, in the course of history, acquired certain representational forms among which are an act of pathological mourning, and we will continue to feel compelled to mourn, Freud suggests, until we modify our attitudes to death—both in the form of a death wish that we have disavowed by turning it into guilt and a death drive we disavow by covering it over with illusions. What fascinates Freud, however, is the manner that this traumatic structure of the unconscious determines not only our rush to destruction but also how it can become a source of creativity and beauty, too.

For, the drives explain why it is man's destiny to desire and be haunted by what he does not have. Perhaps the most painful thing that a person must face is the prospect of his or her own death or the loss of those he loves. Or, as Freud writes in "On War," "Would it not be better to give death the place in reality and in our thoughts that is its due, and bring out the unconscious attitudes to death, which we have hitherto so carefully suppressed, a little more?"[16] But, as he concludes in *Civilization and Its Discontents*:

> Men have gained control over the forces of nature to such an extent that with their help they would have no difficulty in exterminating one another to the last man. They know this, and hence comes a large part of their current unrest, their unhappiness and their mood of anxiety. And now it is to be expected that the other of the two "Heavenly Powers," eternal Eros, will make an effort to assert himself in the struggle with his equally immortal adversary. But who can foresee with what success and with what result?[17]

The next chapter will look at Lacan's idea of the death drive in terms of his idea of the object a, which signifies a fragment of the Real that constantly breaks though the veil of representations and the chains of significations in the Imaginary and Symbolic registers, which covers over the *aporias* of death, and which replaces them with an illusion of transparency. That is, the object a is perhaps an effort to give death some of its due. But this act of giving to death a greater space in consciousness opens up the problem of the sovereignty of lack in the structure of desire. For Lacan, lack is built into the nature of psychic reality and language: representations always are incomplete and leave something out. What I hope to add to this is the notion that the death drive is the agent of the Real that lies outside or beyond the open/closed world of the subject linked to a *jouissance* that is all too often excluded and repressed in the psychic economy.

NOTES

1. Sigmund Freud, *Beyond the Pleasure Principle* in *The Complete Psychological Works of Sigmund Freud*, vol. 18 (New York: W. W. Norton & Co., 1961), 46–47.

2. Freud's neo-Romanticism should never be confused with these reactionary forms of neo-Romanticism. If, for Freud, psychic reality dooms people to experience modern life as *unheimlich*, Freud nowhere roots this *unheimlichkeit* in racial terms, as, for example, Carl Jung does in the thirties and forties, and Freud's early association of the nervous disorders with sexual repression and social hypocrisy is played down after 1920.

3. Freud, *Beyond the Pleasure Principle*, 163.

4. Sigmund Freud, *The Ego and the Id* in *The Complete Psychological Works of Sigmund Freud*, vol. 18 (New York: W. W. Norton & Co., 1960; 1990), 38. Notice that Freud's explanation of the emergence of life eschews the biblical account for an evolutionary one. Life is not something in nature that is sparked by something beyond nature, rather it is a consequence of natural processes.

5. Life develops from, and returns to, death after diverging "ever more widely from its original course of life and . . . (making) ever more complicated *detours*." Freud, *Beyond the Pleasure Principle*, 163. We can see here a typically Freudian combination of Darwinism, with its stress on mechanics (nature as a machine), and Freud's interest in Nature as a life force (as Nature as a spirit or will driving human and natural history forward). Apropos this neo-Romanticism is compatible with a certain (unconventional) reading of Darwin, which argues that Darwin does not turn his back on neo-Romanticism for a mechanistic view of evolution but, instead, reveals the mechanics behind a fundamentally neo-Romantic natural world. In this, his romanticized version of Darwinism, nature functions as a machine in which organisms (discrete organic systems floating in a sea of inorganic compounds) are compelled to change themselves in response to changes in their environment, or become extinct. For what else is natural selection except a mechanism to pass the most adapted or adaptable genes from one generation to the next? Such views remain in opposition to the dominant interpretive tradition that claims that Darwin refuted nature philosophy by showing that variation and change in nature can be explained simply by mechanistic principles. Freud's vitalism (life force and death force), however, posits that a clash of life and death drives lies behind evolution. In his controversial book Robert J. Richards underscores Darwin's possible links to Romanticism when he writes that "Darwin's nature, like that of other German Romantics, exemplified archetypal patterns beneath the wild frenzy of their variations. These patterns gradually change . . .

through the power of a creative nature (*natura naturans*)." Or again: "These laws, taken in the largest sense, being Growth with Reproduction . . . a Ratio of Increase so high as to lead to a Struggle for Life, and as a consequence to Natural Selection, entailing Divergence of Character and the Extinction of lesser improved forms. Thus, from the war of nature, from famine and death, the most exalted object which we are capable of conceiving, namely, the production of the higher animals directly follows." Robert J. Richards, *The Romantic Conception of Life: Science and Philosophy in the Age of Goethe* (Chicago: The University of Chicago Press, 2004), 553.

6. There is also an inherent contradiction built into the pleasure principle as well, which, from the start, Freud speculates, is hopelessly at odds with its own aims and purpose. Thus, he states that the perpetual state of tension we discover in life is due, in large part, to the hopelessly impossible aims of the pleasure principle which are already evident in the earliest experiments in life by Nature.

7. Herman Nunberg and Paul Federn, eds., *Minutes of the Vienna Psychoanalytic Society*, vol. 1 (London: International University Press, Inc., 1962), 175. It is, however, unclear if Stekel develops these suggestions very far.

8. Sigmund Freud, "Dostoevsky and Parricide," in *Character and Culture* (Denver, Colo: Collier Book, 1963), 283–84.

9. Sigmund Freud, *Inhibition, Symptom, and Anxiety* in *The Complete Psychological Works of Sigmund Freud*, vol. 18 (New York: W. W. Norton & Co., 1960; 1990).

10. This object may be what André Green discusses as an object that signifies the "work of the negative" and blank psychosis. In *The Dead Mother* (1999) we find the following: "Decathexis of the object, psychic holes, blank anxiety, depressive emptiness, the dialectics of presence and absence. . . . Instead of an object that has been destroyed there is a psychic hole."

11. Notice what Freud has achieved here. Freud starts out by defining anxiety, as opposed to a fear of something specific, as being generalized, internal, and more or less objectless. But, then, while developing his critique of Rank's birth anxiety, he says that these vague fears of a lost object acquire (in the course of a child's emotional development through the oedipal complex) a certain unconscious link to the fear of castration.

12. Sigmund Freud, *Civilization and Its Discontents* in *The Complete Psychological Works of Sigmund Freud* (New York: W. W. Norton & Co.1961; 1990), 68–69. Earlier in 1919/20, while introducing the idea of a life and death drive to his readers, Freud affirms that "the mind—indeed all life—exists in a state of perpetual conflict and compromise between . . . two trends," that one part of the mind opposes another part of the mind but, more concretely, that impulses to bind and prolong life (Eros) are threatened by destructive urges and by the destructiveness of others too.

13. Freud, *Beyond the Pleasure Principle*, quoted in George Makari, *Revolution in Mind* (New York: HarperCollins, 2008), 317.

14. Apropos this, Freud tells us already, in *Beyond the Pleasure Principle*, that a trauma has as one of its primary characteristics that it compulsively repeats. What gets repeated, in the traumatized unconscious, according to Freud, are a number of

scenes, the most important of which is the oedipal scene, read through the unique life-experiences of each and every subject. Today, it must be said, we are more inclined to see a pre-oedipal scene, too, that exists behind the oedipal scene, and which largely in-forms it. And there are, undoubtedly, other scenes—scenes of birth anxiety, scenes of premature sexual arousal or of premature exposure to death, and so on, that will differ in every person. These other scenes, however, have, as their effect, the same goal of repeating the basic mourning-form for another scene.

15. Even earlier in 1920, Freud writes Ernst Jones: "Can you remember a time so full of death as the present one?" And a few months later, he communicates to Ferenczi in a letter that "the thought of death has not left me." Granted, these comments follow on Sophie's death (and the death of Jones' father and Anton von Freund), but they also reflect ideas and feelings percolating in Freud's unconscious for decades and whose time has, in a manner of speaking, come.

16. Freud writes: "Death can no longer be denied." Freud, "Timely Reflections on War and Death," 185 in Freud, *On Murder, Mourning, and Melancholia* (New York: Penguin Books, 2005).

17. Freud, *Civilization and Its Discontents*, 112.

4

Death and the Other

To the bow is given the name life and its work is death.

—Heraclitus quoted in *The Four Fundamental Concepts of Psychoanalysis*

I plan to review Lacan's concept of death in this chapter. My goal is to treat Lacan as a continuator of Freud's, despite their obvious differences in approach and core assumptions. I will, therefore, ask what Lacan sees when he follows Freud down this rabbit hole and what revelations he makes that may help analysts help their patients confront their erotic death obsessions without being overwhelmed by them. To make the points I want to make will require me to sometimes read Lacan against the grain and to sometimes even read Lacan contra-Lacan, especially in my insistence that we see a connection between the structural role or castration and lack in the formation of the unconscious, on the one hand, and Freud's concept of death on the other hand. Specifically, I will investigate the implications of Lacan's assertion that a fantasy of dying surfaces around the Mirror stage, which the Mirror Stage and the Imaginary register is designed in part to combat—or make disappear—by substituting one experience of death with another experience that reaffirms the image of the body and mind as whole and unfragmented.

Accordingly, I will argue that the Imaginary fantasy of the absent mother is structured by a duality between signs of the mother's presence and absence; and that this duality, which is both conceptual and structural (the concept being constituted by way of a certain structural configuration), tends to become fixated and repeated in the unconscious by the drives when they are not modified by further structural and conceptual development. Lastly, I plan to study the effect of this early death anxiety on development, the neuroses, and on broader cultural issues.

Also, for reasons of economy, I plan to restrict my comments on Lacan to Lacan's middle period, roughly from his public troubles with the SPP, SFP, and the IPA[1] to the founding of Lécole freudienne in 1969. These are fruitful years for Lacan's teaching when he founds his own school, and because it arguably is the theoretical high point of Lacan's teachings during these years, I will use the seminars gathered together in the text *The Four Fundamental Concepts of Psychoanalysis* (1964) as the primary source for my comments in this chapter.

In these seminars, Lacan intervenes in a number of contemporary debates that touch on the historical meaning of humanism and a scientific and anti-humanist revolt against humanism being waged during the fifties and sixties in France by proponents of structuralism and post-structuralism. It is the German Frankfurt school thinker Theodore Adorno who famously says that a person cannot write poetry after Auschwitz. But that is not the only piece of culture shaken by the events of the Holocaust, World War II, and the dawning nuclear age. Humanism, which has been championed since the Renaissance and is closely tied in historiography to the "new method" first applied to study physics and optics in the early modern era, conceives of Mankind as the apex of Nature. For the humanist, Man is a creature unlike any other; consequently, the proper subject of human contemplation should be mankind itself—revealed in its noble aspects and in its struggles to become more noble in bearing and more god-like in action. Yet, after the war, people wonder whether, qua poetry, it is possible to see mankind as noble in aspect and capable of, in the fullness of time, becoming a free and rational being.[2]

This is more than a scream of despair. It is a questioning—this is truer of some post-structuralism than structuralism—of whether rationality and science-centered humanity is entering its maturity or whether the conception of Mankind on which science at least since the Enlightenment is based on a conceptual error. To take just one possible objection, perhaps humanity cannot leave the darkness of mythos and the pathos of death behind so easily without cutting itself off from its own essential nature. Perhaps it is more accurate to say that heretofore history—sometimes seen as a narrative of maturation from superstition to reason and from slavery to freedom—is really a Shakespearean story of blood, murder, and power run amuck, but that a study focusing on the structural relations between elements like kinship patterns or like the elements of language, may produce a truer social science (this also is the era of the Annaliste historians who study history of the long *durée*).

For someone like Lacan, whose version of psychoanalysis has one foot in science and one foot in Heideggerian critique, these are critical questions after the war; and this leads to the question of how Lacan suggests death first appears in the elementary structural relations of the psyche during the mirror stage and what difference exists between the appearance or death in connection to the signifier (or lack) and the drive (libido).

Let us unpack a little of this. In the Imaginary, babies become subjects when their mothers signify to them. Apropos this, I will not repeat the whole narrative of the mirror stage and how the child sees itself in the mirror and then reflected in the gaze of the mother except to say: the position of being a subject emerges first in the give and take of need and desire binding the infant to its mother when the baby responds by generating an image (a fantasy) that signifies the feeling that I (as a subject) need this Other to sustain my identity as a subject. In this sense, the creation of an imago of the subject in the Imaginary parallels the earliest coming together of the logic of needs and desire that bind the baby to the unknown but desired world of the Other. But even before this Imaginary connection occurs, babies already are alienated because they are beings in language. Their mother speaks to them, she already relates to them through the split medium of language where subjects and objects already face each other across an abyss.

But if the baby is born into a "divided" world of language, language remains the only means of reaching out to the other. Therefore, the paradox is that as beings of language, the subject position is forever separated from an object, signifying primal unity and connection, and, yet, language provides people the opportunity of connection so necessary to live, too. One encounters the death drive here, in the desire for an impossible union. To be precise, desire:

> is encountered by the subject in the Other, in the very intimation that the Other makes to him by his discourse. In the intervals of the discourse of the Other, there emerges in the experience of the child something that is radically mappable, namely, He is saying this to me, but what does he want?[3]

The formation of the subject (and formation of the subject of desire), therefore, is marked by a double lack: people are bound to lack by their relation to the drives which are forever partly inaccessible to them and people are bound to lack by what has come to replace an unmediated relation to the drive (libido), that is by the mediation of libido by the logic of language. Hence, humans, says Lacan, are doomed to experience an incompleteness and sense of lack in the fields of sex and language.[4] But Lacan is saying more than this. He also claims that there can be no *jouissance* without lack, and there can be no lack without *jouissance*; and, to go on, beyond Lacan, I would add, there can be no life without death and no Eros without a death drive. And, by the same logic, the subject (which cannot be separated from language, since it emerges by and in language as do the object and the Other that the subject desires) will experience death through this sense of incompleteness at the level of Imaginary (image), the Symbolic (the signifier), and the Real (the subject as the subject of lack). But, as I said, it also experiences this sense of lack in its representation of the subject in relation to both the drive and language since "sex and its significations are always capable of making present the presence of death. . . . On condition that one sees all the sexual drives as articulated at the level of significations in the unconscious, in as much as what they bring out is death—death as a signifier and nothing but a signifier, for can it be said that there is a being-for-death?"[5]

For the entire logic of language as a system of signifiers is about signifying death in the form of lack or absence. Or, what is more often the case, language is a system of signifiers representing the presence of death in the form of lack by not seeing that it is always already there: by acts of denial, repression, and illusion. The inner logic grounding this is summarized by the proposition that unconscious is the discourse of the Other, precisely because it is everything that is desired or feared but not found in the conscious subject.[6]

In a sense, we remain like children, haunted by death that we cannot face because death stalks the subject as its Other through the dualism of presence and absence. One of the forms that presence-absence of death assumes is in the ego's paranoid apprehension of being looked at.

Lacan says that the Imaginary subject is never alone but is always captured by the Other's gaze—just as it seeks to grasp the Other in its gaze. In fact, the whole logic governing the presence and absence of the object of desire is captured in this dance of being seen and not seen, of what is captured and what escapes the gaze. The gaze is a heterogeneous experience for Lacan, a cross between psychological apprehensions of something other (other people, other structures) that seem to lie at the interior of the subject. The gaze, then, is the awareness, partially conveyed in concepts like the uncanny, Althusser's interpolation, spirit-possession, and so on, of being constituted by something other than one's own intentionality, combined with a—however vague—paranoid apprehension. It is like the view of oneself from the other side of the mirror. Lacan says that "we are beings who are looked at"[7] and it is for this reason that people experience themselves as creatures participating in "a speculum mundi,"[8] which at this point we can, by way of commentary, add reflects death and a dread of lack or absence. Developmentally, the mother is the first object signified in the gaze, and, well before the child internalizes the imago of the father, it is she who confronts her child with the discourse of the Other. It is the mother who forms the first gaze peering back into the eyes of her child.

Into every love story a little unhappiness must creep, and Lacan says that it is in the nursery—when the subject, the other, and the ego are just emerging in the child's mind—that death appears in the baby's mind for the first time as a by-product of frustration. Death, says Lacan, is:

> The first object he (the child) proposes for this parental desire whose object is unknown is his own loss—Can he lose me? The fantasy of one's death, of one's disappearance, is the first object that the subject has to bring into play in this dialectic.[9]

Death and the fear of nonbeing then appear at the moment when the child becomes a subject, at the moment, that is, when the child links the image in the mirror of himself to the signification of the mother, at the same time the child is also able to conceive the idea of the mother's absence and hence of its own nonbeing (non-signification).[10]

Unfortunately for our little hero, things are amiss from the start and the world seems out of kilter in some mysterious ways. The problem initially is one of expectations. Lacan may not have emphasized this, but the almost wholly narcissistic baby, with only the vaguest awareness of the world of the other at first, treats the mother as an extension of its own demands and wishes. Whether one believes, like Freud, in a state of primary narcissism at birth or one believes, like Michael Balint, that babies are object-relating from birth, the mother is not yet an other in the mature sense of being another person with her own desires and intentionality that are different from the baby's wishes and desires. Rather, she is still only a shadow-other, a limb of the child's desire; and her consistent failures are at first perplexing and enraging to the child. He treats her like a tyrant would treat a slave and he cannot understand why this limb-mother seems to posses a divided mind. And, although he does not have the conceptual or linguistic ability to formulate the problem this way yet, his reaction speaks for him. He acts as if he wants to say: why is the limb-mother so inconsistent? She dreams of work and her husband and other family members all of whom pull her away when she should give her full attention to me![11]

So begins the child's recurring experience of the mother as an ambivalent object that can be the source of comfort and satisfaction at one moment and starvation and lack in the next moment. And, as I just said, it is into this unhappy love affair, this mixed bag, that death appears for the first time as a sign in the head of our little hero—and it is here that it will stay for the rest of his life as a sign of lack and absence of the mother or a surrogate. Apropos this, consider the dream first reported by Freud in *The Interpretation of Dreams*, and discussed by Lacan in *The Four Fundamental Concepts of Psychoanalysis*, in which a dead child returns to his mourning father to complain that he is burning. Here, transposed into an oedipal dream, lies another Imaginary scene about the mother's non-presence—when the father says in effect—"my son is no longer here!" Thus, he repeats the child's anxiety of having lost the mother. And the son responds—"father, you are not beside me while I am burning!"[12]

Thus, while the male noun "he" in the above-mentioned quote may suggest Lacan is only speaking of the loss of the father and the oedipal crisis, a closer reading reveals that this is not the case. It shows rather that the oedipal complex repeats another prior scene. But this other scene has different characters engaged in a different drama where what is possibly lost is not the penis-phallus but existence itself.

It is the mother to whom the child first turns his fear that he may die; and, consequently, the mother will be the first other with whom the child will bargain to delay death, and whose actions and desires he will try to control and capture (seduce if you will) in order to protect himself from possibly being abandoned to death. Thus begins "the aim of catching the *jouissance* of the Other"[13] which, Lacan says, forces the child to recognize, "in so far as the other intervenes . . . that there is a *jouissance* beyond the pleasure principle," i.e., that there is a *jouissance* of the other to take in account the struggle to find pleasure and to stay alive.[14]

The mother—qua other—therefore is connected to the child's earliest experience of lack and defeat. As Lacan says: "The desire of the Other is apprehended by the subject in that which does not work, in the lacks of the discourse of the Other."[15] And to Lacan's idea I want to add the point that on the level of the drives, death drives are being mobilized and defenses are being mustered that produce the sorts of eroticized death drives that we have seen before. In these situations, however, they appear as eroticized death drives aiming at the imago of the mother's absence or presence. Given this, the child may experience a painful sensation of presence rather than no presence at all; and, all things considered, the same child may submit to a painful sensation that is known before one that is unknown because lack, at this point, is connected to a fear of non-existence. The fear of being lost is only transferred onto the father and the phallus at a later date, and the threat of castration (which the Symbolic registry is designed to police and regulate) is, therefore, a later developmental version of the threat that the mother will lose the child by not being present—an association that leads to the even stranger association of the mother-phallus![16]

Thus, just as Abraham substitutes the ram for Isaac, the child substitutes the phallus for the mother who (in the oedipal complex) has become taboo. But it is in relation to the mother that the child first experiences apprehension and the fear of death upon worrying whether she is present or absent.

A link, therefore, can be deduced between the developmentally earlier fear of dying (non-presence) and the developmentally later oedipal anxiety of being castrated. For, from an early age, the mind associates presence (of the breast, the mother, a transitional object, the phallus) with the avoidance of primitive anxiety. Apropos this, the fort/da game, which Lacan refers to in many places in *The Four Fundamental Concepts of Psychoanalysis*, stages an encounter between the mother and child as a game of absence and presence. This game of lost and found (Lacan calls it a game of "here and there") allows the child to lessen the anxiety caused by the mother's absence. What is more, the game gets transposed in part from anxiety to speech. Thus, the mother's going is followed in the game by the child's commentary: "oooooo." Similarly, when Freud's grandson pulls back on the string and makes this symbol of his mother return to its place, he sighs with a gleeful "aaa." In this, Freud's grandson shows the power of language to transpose an anxiety or drive, as well as the early entanglement of speech and magical thinking to reduce unpleasantness. Also, based on what we now know, it is not just the mother who is represented as being "here and there." It also is the child who is being lost and found with each tug of the string as the mother magically disappears and reappears. The game, therefore, puts a *petit mort* in play, a little auto- auto-de-fe, which will resurface in separation anxiety, stranger anxiety, the fear of the dark, the wish for invisible friends, and monsters hiding under the bed, too.[17] Later, the same game of making present plays a role in some kinds of collecting, and possibly some eating disorders as well.

Among the implications this suggests is the idea that food defines the oral drive less well than does the child's search to incorporate the lost object since "no food will ever satisfy the oral drive, except by circumventing the eternally lacking object."[18] One implication of this that Lacan does not mention is that, to resolve infantile conflicts, a child has to modify not only the relation between his superego and his ego's fear of death, but the relation between his ego and his unconscious desires as well.[19] An argument can, therefore, be made that the two developmental ways of being in the world that Lacan calls the Imaginary and the Symbolic are different, structured reactions to the same basic fear of the Real. These sometimes take the form of a defense against absence of the mother and at other times it takes the form of a defense against castration anxiety. But, in either case, the constructed reality is a defense against the fear of dying or being irretrievably damaged by hostility vis-à-vis the Other.

At this point in the chapter, I want to step back from what I have been discussing one moment in order to provide some brief clarifications. The first clarification concerns the way the representation of death is multi-valient.

What this means is that the principal psychological anxieties I have stressed so far (those surrounding the fear of the absence or loss of the mother as a repetition of the loss or nonappearance of the primal object) represent only the primary representation-anxiety of death at the Imaginary level. Lacan, however, is perhaps best known for his discussion of the representation of death at the Symbolic level which he associates with the signification of the "dead father" and the creation of the Law of the Father signifier that underlies the symbolic order. I therefore want to spend a little time clarifying the difference between the Imaginary fear of losing the mother and the Symbolic (castration) fears connected to the identification with the signifier for the dead father. I then want to infer a little bit on the relation between these two signifiers as sources of anxiety of and defenses against death in the register of the Real, which I take to be best signified by the Lacanian concept of the object a and which can be incompletely described as the appearance (in the form of an object) of something that signifies the presence of the absent primal object—that is that represents the subject's apprehensive intuition within the field of language of the Thing that is desired but cannot be represented in any way; a Thing that Lacan defines variously, but which can roughly be linked to the fact that humans are *parletre*, speaking beings, who, as such, remain forever cut off from the natural world (hence a part of themselves to the extent that they are part of the natural world) in any but the most mediated forms.

In a book on the work of André Green, Gregorio Kohon defines Lacan's idea of the dead father in the following manner. He says that it represents "the continuity of the previous generations through the superego (the Law of the father)."[20] In other words, Lacan is following Freud in associating the creation of the Symbolic order with the defensive reaction to two things: first the son's own impulses to murder and take the place of the father and, second, the son's guilt and anxiety for having done the deed. Lacan says as much when he asks: "Do we not see, behind this, the emergence of that which forced Freud to find in the myths of the death of the father the regulation of desire?—The death of the father being a shelter against the threat of castration."[21] The Symbolic order, which Lacan associates with the general structure of libido within a logical system of linguistic signs and symbols, is then directly linked to the defensive anxiety of giving into one's death drive and the guilt associated with having already committed the deed. And, I would add, that the anxiety (this is not anxiety as Lacan defines it in his seminars) of the death drive lies behind the entire development of mental and cultural life, which assumes the strange beginning in an identification with a ghost (a dead father) who: "became stronger than the living one had been—for events took the course we so often see them follow in human affairs to this day. What had up to then been prevented by his actual existence was thenceforward prohibited by the sons themselves, in accordance with the psychological procedure so familiar to us in psychoanalyses under the name of 'deferred obedience?'"[22] One can say, then, that the whole Symbolic order is a system of substitutions for, and signifiers signifying, something we do not want to remember and cannot recall: the lost primal object.

In a sense, the relation to a lost primal object that lies behind the Symbolic order (that the logic of language itself is all about) precedes the emergence of the Imaginary since it is already implied in the mother's desire as she looks and handles her baby. And, given this preexisting reality, it is no wonder that when the child enters the Imaginary and begins to formulate a world for itself around images (words will soon follow) it will discover this same longing for the lost desire of the other to be at the foundation of everything. That is, that the child's earliest Imaginary relations to itself, its body, and to its mother will be informed by this logic such that the child's whole calculus (his whole gamble on life) turns on the problem of fulfilling the desire of the Other (the Mother) so that the Mother will not leave him (that is so that the mother will fulfill the infant's desire).

On the other hand, Lacan comments in *Écrits* on the affinity between "the themes of the father and death" in Freud's work in this way. He says that an affinity exists between "the appearance of the signifier of the father, as author of the Law" and "the murder of the Father—thus showing that if this murder is the fruitful moment of debt through which the subject binds himself for life to the Law, the Symbolic Father is, in so far as he signifies this Law, the dead Father."[23] And, Lacan adds elsewhere in the *Écrits*, when speaking about how the Law or castration anxiety (the fear of absence and lack) is the actual subject that lies behind the entire chain of signifiers in the Symbolic register, that any signification is only possible in relation to that "dummy" the dead father.

In other words, both the Symbolic logic of the signifier (as a subject for another signifier) and the Imaginary relations to death are efforts to replace the emptiness of lacking (the dead father, the absented mother) with a fantasy or a substitute form of satisfaction that is never able to quite cover over the hole left by loss: that is the pathos of being the *parletre*, the speaking subject.

And although Lacan does not say this, failure to resolve the association between absence-death and castration-guilt only strengthens the paranoid ego and its defenses, which, in turn, support the development of neurotic and psychotic solutions to unresolved infantile sexual and aggressive conflicts; and a vicious circle can develop in which a fantasy of death leads to defenses against absence, while, alternatively, a feeling of absence will trigger representations, wishes, and anxieties of dying or murder.

Without claiming any nosological significance, we can organize people's attitudes toward death as falling into one of three categories for heuristic purposes even though these do not appear in Lacan. The first is composed of the traumatized. This consists of people who are in the midst of conscious or preconscious trauma that they continue to repeat over and over despite their obvious distress. All these people share two characteristics. They are victims of a trauma and they are obsessed by images of death, dying, or loss. This will include Holocaust survivors and their children who are themselves often traumatized, veterans, those who suffer from major depressions and are constantly thinking about their loss and the death of parents or loved ones, people with anxiety who constantly fear someone they love may die or are unable to overcome the death of a loved one. One man who I see, for example, survived being a soldier for six years with no serious neurosis despite having mild anxiety attacks since he was a child. But when his sister, nephew, and best friend all died within six months he fell into a deep depression in which all his anxiety about death—from childhood, from the war, and from his more recent losses—haunted him. A second group includes the non-traumatized people who, nevertheless, show signs of being obsessed by death or death anxiety. This group includes many neurotics, and those who are vulnerable to developing a neurosis because of unresolved fixations from childhood that turn on death and death anxiety. Some people from this group carry what André Green calls a dead mother or a dead father inside them. Often, they will not show signs of a disturbance until some external shock—such as the death of their parents—brings all the conflicts that they thought they had resolved about death and dying back to the forefront of their minds. Another patient lived with his mother with no problems after his father, who he internalized as a cruel man, died. But when his mother died suddenly he too became deeply depressed. When he came into treatment with me he, after just a few preliminary sessions, reported he had a dream in which he is being buried alive by a man in a white robe and a man in a black robe. He is terrified, he says, in the dream, but he seems strangely excited when he repeats it to me in session. He adds that he had had the same dream when his mother died but had forgotten about it since. In his associations to the dream, which continue for many sessions, he eventually reveals that the man in the dream being buried alive is not himself but his brother who died in the navy and was buried by soldiers in white and black uniforms. And we can feel certain that his brother stands in, as a replacement, for his cruel father, who he would like to see in the grave a second time—the apprehension reflects his guilt or fear of reappraisal. A third group includes those who have sublimated their childhood fears of dying and developed mature attitudes toward death and loss by dint of an analysis or luck.

Resolving these childhood death anxieties, of course, is just one dimension of the cure. But, by the same token, an analysis that heals depression or anxiety, for example, without addressing the patient's infantile attitudes toward death and dying will remain incomplete, and may lead nowhere. For, alongside libidinal development, self development, object-relations maturation, and improved interpersonal relations, the psyche has to develop new attitudes toward death too.

But only the analysand can give them up. The analyst cannot do this for her. But, the analyst's attitude can play a decisive role in creating what Winnicott called a proper setup for the cure to occur. To reduce the power of the ego's omnipotence, Lacan suggests that the analyst frustrate the analysand by not giving in to his or her demands. This "active therapy" first practiced by Ferenczi and Rank is supposed to overcome resistance and stir up the unconscious communications. In this regard, it bears comparison to Klein's interpreting the unconscious content directly to her child analysands in age-appropriate language. In both cases, resistance and other defenses are disregarded more than made the focus of interpretation and working through as they are in the very different therapies of Wilhelm Reich and Anna Freud.

But, while it is sometimes helpful to join the unconscious desire directly, it has been my experience that too much frustration arouses too much anxiety when working with primitive death anxiety; so the analyst must resist the wish to communicate unconscious desires simply to relieve his own psychic tensions. If one interprets the unconscious or tries to let it speak (I strongly recommend the latter more than the former), one always has to pay respect to the defenses which can guide the analyst to know how much unconscious material, and how much anxiety, the analysand can tolerate.

In other words, while working toward making the unconscious conscious and helping the analysand put their death anxieties and fantasies into speech acts which can be altered, the analyst's primary job is to monitor the analysand's anxiety level and never let it rise too fast, since the first obligation of the analyst is to protect the analysand as they work toward the truth of their unconscious desires.

In an article on group destructive resistances, the Modern group analyst Leslie Rosenthal recalls that it was Freud who:

> offered the first clue that resistance was an immature way of functioning and provided the basis for the subsequent recognition that resistance phenomena are identified with the defenses called upon by the ego to maintain emotional equilibrium and to ensure psychological survival.[24]

Lacan, of course, describes the ego and its functioning differently than Rosenthal. For Lacan, the ego is a paranoid system that represses the subject of desire and the knowledge that the subject is split or divided. But, bearing this in mind, we can still say that, exactly so, the struggle the analysis stirs up will be met by resistances, and among these will be a resistance to modifying the analysand's relation to their death drive, often by the unconscious projection of primitive anxiety and death wishes into the analyst. Therefore, a second goal, while working with his analysand's death anxieties, is to set limits for the analysand when he or she is acting out a treatment resistant behavior.

At other times, the analyst needs to get out of the way of the analysand's communications and let him develop an idealized or a hostile transference. Transference has come to mean all the feelings the analysand has for the therapist. But, in the sense I want to stress, the transference has a more technical meaning. It is a form of repetition and resistance formed between the analyst and analysand, but a particularly intense repetition of the analysand's errors and defensiveness about knowing the structure of his desire, the nature of his relation to the other, and his own history.

By proceeding in this way, the analyst allows the transference to develop and at the same time introduces something new into the transference relationship, namely he introduces his non-judgmental position, thereby guaranteeing the psychoanalysis does not just replicate the old encounter, but creates the conditions by which the analysand can experience a different outcome.

The Modern psychoanalyst Stanford Bazilian published an article in the nineties in which he warns the analyst against giving into a destructive countertransference reaction and says that the outcome of an analysis may depend on the analyst's controlling his aggression so that he does no harm. This becomes especially critical when working with an analysand's unconscious death anxieties. This is not anything that has not been gone over before, but it bears repeating. The strain that the analyst is placed under may elicit their own counter-transference reactions that have to be monitored and held in check.

This, however, does not mean that the analyst inhibits his own aggression. Often aggression cannot be avoided and, all things considered, if aggressive feelings emerge it is better for the analysis, and the analyst, to have them and silently explore them rather than let them adversely affect the analysis. But if the negative feelings become too overwhelming, if they become a counter-transference treatment destructive behavior, than besides speaking to a colleague the analyst can try to find something he or she can admire in the analysand's most irritating behavior. For example, when the analysand seems full of destructive and excessive rage, the analyst may admire the analysand's ability to feel fury. Or, if the analysand is unbearably depressed, the analysand may admire his analysand's depth of feeling.[25] But this cannot be simply a trick. It must be genuine admiration or it will not work.

Finally, an analysis does not exist in a black box somewhere apart from society. That kind of thinking is associated with experimental psychology that controls for as many external variables as possible. An analysis is something that occurs in a private office, but it arouses all the Symbolic and Imaginary images and fantasies that have gone into the individual's whole life story. This is a story in which the subject of desire of the analysand has been buried by the pressure of the Symbolic order and the nature of the ego's paranoia (which often is a social paranoia, too). And, so long as the paranoid ego dictates how the subject reacts to dying, life remains a sort of Darwinian battleground of anxiety and unrelenting rivalry, where the dragon must be slain or rivalry prematurely ended.

The epistophilic drive is especially linked to the child's early fear of dying, since it is this fear that compels the child to want to know the desire of the mother so as to keep her near. From the start, the epistophilic drive is both stimulated and distorted by this fear, when, for instance, the child disavows that the mother is absent to offset his anxiety that he will die. Manic and omnipotent defenses help the child keep the other in its place by second-guessing: "What does he want (from me)?" [26]

The essential point is that when the child asks "What does the Other want from me?" this is the moment when the child bites the apple and the whole life history of the subject and the ego's misperceptions of its own subjectivity are set in motion. The child must know the desire of the Other to relieve its fear of dying; but the child cannot know. The child's response to this conundrum can best be described, in a monstrous parody of Hegel, as a long dialectic evolution from error (ego) to the truth of the unconscious desire of the analysand (cure) which is, at the Symbolic level, tied to the triumph of science and, at the individual level, to the triumph of psychoanalysis.

I already have alluded to Hegel's master-slave dialectic and the Heideggerian critique of Western thought and rationality, and even how Lacan may be situated in regards to a French Nietzschean elitist and transgressive philosophy. I now will draw some of these points out a little more in relation to death.

Uniting Lacan's scientism and his Heideggerianism is a profound longing to uncover a deeper truth of desire. At the same time, Lacan is interested in the structural inhibitions to arriving at the truth of desire which is always the truth of this or that subject. Lacan does not frame the split at the heart of the subject as a Nietzschean discourse of heroic revolt and decentered subjectivity, if for no other reason than Lacan insists more than Nietzsche's French followers that subjectivity follows linguistic rules structuring and defining the forms of subjectivity in every era, and, by these laws, rebellion can be as much a flight from the truth of desire into omnipotent egoism as a liberation. Apropos this, there is a scene in the novel *Le bleu du ciel* (1935), translated as *The Blue of Noon*, by George Bataille (the novel explores the inhibitions to the hero's quest for a Nietzschean, sacred experience that shatters the categories of "normal experience," and that summarizes this state of blockage and revolt wonderfully well); it is an image of a farmer standing—waiting—in his fields for the storm to come that may very well destroy him. The ecstatic shattering of the doors of perception are all for Bataille, and the destruction of the subject—nothing. But, Lacan is far too much of a secularist to be swept up by Bataille's form of identification of the subject with excess which is nothing than the search for a form of the sacred suitable to modern life. He does, however, conceive of psychoanalysis as an instrument for unveiling the truth of the unconscious, allowing the subject to discover the true structure of its desire and, therefore, unveil what the British independent Christopher Bollas calls one's own idiom, grounded in a truer understanding of one's divided nature and one's own history.

Lacan's goal is not to unlock sacred energy encrusted behind the rigid modern masks of rationalism and consciousness, but to lessen the defenses and illusions keeping the subject in a state of error about its own desire, about the fact that the subject is irremediably split, and about the realization that a part of being will always be missing, "not there,"[27] and subject to disturb the sleep of consciousness.

Consider, for example, Lacan's discussion of Han's Holbein's anamorphosis painting "The Ambassadors." When looking at the painting frontally, Lacan informs his seminar, the viewer perceives two ambassadors flanking symbols of the vanity of life. This conventional view of political power works by staging an encounter between an image and a viewer of the image whose meanings are preestablished in the Symbolic order. As a representation of the Symbolic whose power and presence are guaranteed by its ability to repress or police the signs of castration and death, the painter highlights what should appear in the viewer's field of perceptions and consciousness. But when one looks at the picture awry, Lacan says, one sees a death's skull. In other words, the conventional image that the viewer is supposed to see according to the rules of Renaissance optics, the new Cartesian perspectivism, and a certain Christian moral iconography, is being subverted by a view from the other side—by death.

The painting or the painter of the painting, in other words, stages an encounter between two perceptions: one displays the traditional signs of power and vanity and the other is the repressed sign of death and nothingness. Together, they reveal the split nature of the subject, revealed, Lacan says, in the appearance of an object a in the field of perception. The object a, says Lacan, is linked to what is lacking, to "that part of himself that the individual loses at birth, and which may serve to symbolize the most profound lost object."[28] The appearance of the object a signals the presence of "the subject as annihilated," that it signals "the death head that signifies our own nothingness."[29] It permits the subject to glimpse the inassimilable thing which should not appear in the subject's field of perception—signs of castration, death, nothingness, and absence (non-presence).

But we must not overlook the obvious. The object a is exactly what Lacan says it is. It is a signifier of an object. But, more importantly is an object that signifies the nonrepresentational. It is the signifier of nothingness or the paradoxical appearance in the positive chain of signifiers of negation, the hole in all meanings that overflows and acts like a well sucking into its void all the significations of desire. Thus, this object must be differentiated from the positive sorts of objects that Melanie Klein and others mention are introjected and used to build up the ego's object relations world. One can make a rough analogy that goes like this, however: the object a is to positive internal objects as castration and lack associated with the lost primal object are to the chain of signifiers that seek to fill in the gap it has left behind. At the same time, the object a should be differentiated from the Big A: the Law of the Father or castration that makes the Symbolic chain of significations meaningful. Also, it hardly needs saying that the object a is not the same as a natural object since it is by its very nature a creation of the transformation language has wrought to the human experience of its own subjectivity, its own desire, its own experience of *jouissance* and satisfaction, and its own experience of its objects (the typical illustration of the object transformed by language and desire is the Imaginary object the child encounters of itself as it peers into the mirror). The key to these objects is that they cannot satisfy desire completely. Or, as Lacan writes, the subject makes of himself an object "by displaying himself before the mirror, (but) he could not be satisfied with it" (this lack of satisfaction being the hallmark of objects in the human world).[30]

Thus, the object a is the object for the subject that paradoxically signifies lack, the failure of the object and desire; and what can we call that but the work of the death drive? For we can say without being too far off the mark that the object a is the trace of the death and libido drive that appears in the form of a positive object that the subject desires. It is the object through whose presence the "work of the negative" appears in consciousness. Or, to say this differently, it is the object through which the subject comes face to face with the failure of desire that Lacan elsewhere associates with the Real.

As such, it is not an object found in the natural world but is a sort of logical linguistic place holder for the paradoxical place of negation in language. It is the thing that constantly keeps positive objects from being truly satisfying. And we can say it is never really there, being in essence more akin to a ghost than a positive thing in that it signifies in the realm of positive objects the trace of the lost primal object that can never be found again.

If the object a is more a logical place holder for nothingness than it is a positivity, then we are obviously wasting our time searching for "it" or even trying to nail down a proper definition of it. For, "it" always escapes from positive forms, being nothing but the trace in the world of object of the thing that makes all objects unsatisfactory in the end. However, I want to stress the similarity between this and the Freudian notions of the death drive. Thus, the object a marks the return to consciousness of "some primal separation, some self-mutilation induced by the very approach of the real."[31] It sticks in the craw, in a manner of speaking because, says Lacan, the object a "cannot be swallowed" and "gets stuck in the gullet of the signifier."[32] The object a is something that the ego chokes on, something that is "inscribed in the ego as non-ego, negation, splitting off of the ego."[33]

The message being conveyed by Holbein's painting, therefore, ultimately is not that everything is vanity when power lies outside of the presence of God, which would be the moral iconography of the Symbolic order, but that all is vanity because power and presence are thinkable only in relation to castration, death, and lack—the very knowledge that the Imaginary and the Symbolic try to repress. The object a, therefore, can at one moment lay stress to the sovereign moment and at the next to the moment of revolution—the point being that both are bound to one another by the very structure of desire that the object a unveils to our consciousness. Thus, the object a can appear anywhere, in theatrical performers staging monstrously stylized rituals marked by exaggerated violent gestures that amaze and seduce audiences, even in mimicry, where the signs function as a warning to the other to stay away! (I can castrate you!) or as a seduction, enticing the other to come closer. It can signify Otherness, it can be linked to an impulse to keep a threatening idea or image outside of the areas of consciousness and perception, or it can be a drive to maintain a thought, idea, or behavior in the forefront of consciousness so as to not think of something unthinkable; but, life is unthinkable, too, without death, and, for this reason, death can also be put to use to regulate the encounter between other people and the world qua Others.[34] But, whatever is being signified, it always returns to the meaning Freud stresses when he makes castration anxiety the price people pay to be returned to the bosom of the Symbolic.[35]

What then is the narrative being staged by the object a except a sign whose prototypes are to be found in Saussure's linguistics and in the infant's anxiety that the mother may not be present? The object a brings this whole encounter into the field of perception as a differential relationship of presence and absence, here and not here. The impact of the Other and the influence of linguistics are so inextricably linked, as Lacan expresses it: "the subject determined by language and speech . . . begins in the locus of the Other, in so far as it is there that the first signifier emerges" as to be inseparable.[36] We, ultimately, have no way of knowing for certain whether language or the encounter with the mother is the first or more basic encounter—except to say that, from the perspective of the *long durée*, the child is already borne into a Symbolic whose rules of discourse are preset, but, from the perspective of the individual, the encounter with the mother is more fundamental. But in both encounters, the child's response to death and the Other is the essential thing—just as Freud describes in *Beyond the Pleasure Principle* (1920); that is, life is a story of Eros' struggle to delay death and keep the death drive at bay.

What do we do with death? Do we freeze time in a kind of eternal presence or should we forget like the Egyptians allegedly forgot the founder of monotheism and the Jews forgot the original murdered Moses? Or, do we accept loss and start living from there? It is one of the ironies of life that Lacan may have learnt from Kojeve's strange "communist" reading of Nietzsche's "last Man" and Hegel's "end of History," that so long as the fear of dying is left unmodified, the subject will be brow-beaten and dominated by a paranoid ego. History and the Spirit, it seems, may need psychoanalysis to overcome the infantile fear of dying and non-presence by transforming anxiety into speech acts.

Still, a person can find unlimited reasons why moderating one's infantile fantasy of presence is a bad idea. The way forward, however, demands a willingness to admit that one is mortal, that one day we will be—nothing, and that our longing to live is impossible outside of death. It is an old idea: read Homer, but without necessarily buying its promotion of a tragic heroic response. In the next chapter, I will look at how we can incorporate death into an ethic based on an awareness of the individual's place in the chain binding each of us to the generations who come before and the generations who follow us and to those who live in this world with us.

NOTES

1. Paris Psychoanalytic Society, The French Society of Psychoanalysis (Lagache's group), and International Psychoanalytic Associations.

2. This is one of the aims of secular humanism which is not the same thing as Christian humanism. American consumerism is another reaction to postwar anomie.

3. Lacan, *The Four Fundamental Concepts of Psychoanalysis*, trans. Alan Sheridan (New York: W. W. Norton & Co., 1998) 214.

4. Lacan, *The Four Fundamental Concepts*, 204.

5. Lacan, *The Four Fundamental Concepts*, 257. And finally: "Analytic experience substitutes the search by the subject, not of the sexual complement, but of a part of himself, lost forever, that is constituted by the fact that he is only a sexed living being, and that he is no longer immortal." Lacan, *The Four Fundamental Concepts*, 205.

6. Foucault of course does not argue this precisely since for him it is equally important to show how madness and the contemporary relation between reason and death are products of historical structures of modernity more than a putative *drive*, which Foucault would consider atavistic return to an idea of biology and naturalism. We, however, find this too extreme a position to adopt.

7. Lacan, *The Four Fundamental Concepts*, 75.

8. Lacan, *The Four Fundamental Concepts*, 75. This is not exactly the same notion as, for example, Foucault's discussion of a medical gaze in *The Birth of Clinic* or the panopticon in *Discipline and Punish* or even the one Merleau-Ponty mentions is a part of the structure of a phenomenological experience.

9. Lacan, *The Four Fundamental Concepts*, 257.

10. The mother then is the first Other. She holds a power over me, she exercises a kind of seduction, and she is threatening to me as well. She is not simply a sign of all that is "not subject" but someone with whom the subject is always in some kind of extreme *encounter*. The subject only exists in relation to what it is not and wants and the Other only assumes meaning in relation to a subject that is its other. One way Lacan investigates this encounter in *The Four Concepts* is by developing the concept of the object a. The object a, Lacan says, establishes "an essential encounter—an appointment to which we are always called with a real that eludes us." When he says the "real" in this context he may just as well have said Other. We will have more to say on the object a in the body of this chapter later on. Also, the superego, a concept Lacan disavows, highlights the bipolarity of the Other as being inside and outside (just as in theology God or evil is both inside and outside the person). But it does so by using psychological categories like introjections and identification. Thus the superego is described in *The Ego and the Id* by Freud as outside, given that it stands over the ego as the internal representative of Symbolic power and morality. At the same time, the superego lies inside in that it is internalized and made an object of identification by the ego. But Lacan repudiates the structural model as formalistic (a strange criticism for the author of the mathemes) in part to substitute his own ideas about the encounter between subject and the other in its place. Winnicott proposed a transitional space to convey a sense of an object that is co-created by mother and infant (encounter). Lacan shows how the subject and the object are co-created by being placed in relation to signs of lack and desire.

11. There once was a book called *The God That Failed* about Communism. In the Imaginary, the mother appears in the child's fantasy as like a goddess who is prone to failure because she cannot satisfy all the child's demands or, alternatively, the child cannot satisfy or even know all her desires. This initiates, in my opinion, a sort of game about its relation to the maternal body where the child tries to disavow lack and then later castration anxiety.

12. Lacan, *The Four Fundamental Concepts*, 58. Dass das Kind an seinem Bette steht, that the child is near his bed, ihn am Arme fasst, takes him by the arm and whispers to him reproachfully, und ihm vorwurfsvoll zurant: Vater, siehst du denn nicht, Father, can't you see, dass ich verbrenne, that I am burning?

13. Jean-Michel Rabaté makes the useful clarification that *jouissance* "translates Bataille's concepts of waste, expenditure, erotic excess, and transgression" in Jean-Michel Rabaté, "Lacan's turn to Freud," in *The Cambridge Companion to Lacan* (Cambridge: Cambridge University Press, 2006), 38.

14. Lacan, *The Four Fundamental Concepts*, 183–84.

15. Lacan, *The Four Fundamental Concepts*, 257. There is a certain theological discourse exemplified by the story of Job in which what is at stake is the gap, the incomprehensibility and inequality in the encounter between God and man. Psychoanalysis suggests this originates as a problem first in the nursery.

16. The oedipal complex tries to obscure this.

17. We also can see how a fantasy of dying is integrated within the mind's normal processes of keeping disturbing ideas (such as I will die if I am neglected by the Other) from entering the field of perception and consciousness. Also, we can, by and by, see how the belief in immortality is to the fear of dying as the belief in a father in heaven is to a fear of castration. In both, an unconscious infantile conflict becomes displaced and projected onto an image that basically negates the original disturbing idea.

18. Lacan, *The Four Fundamental Concepts*, 180.

19. The development of libido from pre-genital to genital love, for example, and the development of object relations from narcissism to object love are all affected by the maturation or fixation in childhood attitudes toward death.

20. Gregorio Kohon, "Preface," in *The Dead Mother, The Work of André Green*, ed. Gregorio Kohon (London: Routledge, 1999) p. 5.

21. Lacan, *The Four Fundamental Concepts*, 27.

22. Sigmund Freud, *Totem and Taboo*, Standard Editions, vol. XIII (London: Routledge, 1950)

23. Jacques Lacan, "On a Question Preliminary to Any Possible Treatment of Psychosis," in *Écrits*, trans. Alan Sheridan (London: Routledge, 1977).

24. Leslie Rosenthal, "The Resolution of Group-Destructive Resistance in Modern Group Analysis," *Modern Psychoanalysis*, 30B (2005), 243.

25. In treatment with regressed patients, the analysand must be made to feel he or she can use the analyst without fearing retaliation in the early stages of the analysis and in those later portions of the analysis when the patient has become severely regressed and therefore full of destructive death drives and fantasies of a violent and deadly nature. In particular during these regressed phases the analysand will be inclined—and must be allowed—to use the analyst to repeat their most primitive fantasies that turn on the linkage between death and desire that was established in the first years of life. At other times, the analyst has to allow the analysand to use the analyst to distract him or herself from this fantasy association of desire and death. And, since death and desire are points on a continuum, the analyst may appear at other times in the preconscious

of the patient in the transference as an object signifying death or as an object that the subject must repel to avoid the appearance of fantasies of death. At other times the analyst may become something akin to the self-object and act as a cornerstone against death.

26. Lacan, *The Four Fundamental Concepts*, 257. In the Imaginary, this questioning of the Other is so I can capture the mother's desire and in the Symbolic so that I can submit to the Law of the dead Father and so enter the Symbolic order.

27. Both Nietzsche and Heidegger had already analyzed this flight from the world of time and change into an illusory world of changeless essences, and consequently both become essential figures legitimating this post-structural critique of both structuralism and humanism—although both remain suspected characters for their (very different) connections to National Socialism. Heidegger in particular associates a subject's Being with a "heroic" and "lonely" existence open to potentially limitless numbers of ways of existing, already implicitly calling for the death of the humanist subject in *Being and Time* (1927). Thus Heidegger stressed in *Being and Time* that something makes people turn away from Being so the mind is distracted by entertainment and other superficialities. "Distraction" and entertainment carry the same weight as Freud's analytic concept of repression—both lead the subject to resist the encounter with Otherness (defined differently as the unconscious for Freud and Being for Heidegger). Heidegger was struck however by the fact that people prefer "inauthentic lives" when such a life frees them from the burden of remaining open to the constantly changing possibilities of Being—that is they feel more at home in a certain world that is totally at odds with Being. Sometimes however, Heidegger added, people do open themselves to the unknown possibilities of Being and what happens is that they feel *vertigo* when their normal existential frames of reference are momentarily swept away. Heidegger therefore proposes that there is a sort of metaphysical *angst*, just as Freud argued people resist making the unconscious conscious. For just as Freud wished to lessen resistances to bringing the unconscious into the field of consciousness, Heidegger wanted to overcome whatever distracted philosophers from facing the problem of Being and of bringing it into the field of conscious perception (thinking).

28. Lacan, *The Four Fundamental Concepts*, 198.

29. Sartre and other continental philosophers also applied Phenomenology to a variety of existential problems such as the meaning of death and the problem of inauthenticity in ways that could only interest psychoanalysts like Lacan. See Lacan, *The Four Fundamental Concepts*, 88.

30. Lacan, "The Function and Field of Speech and Language in Psychoanalysis," *Écrits*, trans. Alan Sheridan.

31. Lacan, *The Four Fundamental Concepts*, 83.

32. Lacan, *The Four Fundamental Concepts*, 270.

33. Lacan, *The Four Fundamental Concepts*, 245.

34. "The effect of mimicry is camouflage, in the strictly technical sense. It is not a question of harmonizing with the background," but of appearing "like an ideal ego to the other." Lacan, *The Four Fundamental Concepts*, 99.

35. In this respect, the object a resembles latent thoughts that come into perception through the construction of a dream, a ghost from the other side that ties us in knots. We are forced to see ourselves from the perspective of what the Symbolic rejects as a sign of castration, as inassimilable (cannot be incorporated into the chain of signification of desire and speech), rejected, repressed, distorted, and masked.

36. Lacan, *The Four Fundamental Concepts*, 99.

5

Death and the Chain of Life

> The life of Spirit is not the life that shrinks from death and keeps itself untouched by devastation, but rather the life that endures. . . . Spirit is this power only by looking the negative in the face, and tarrying with it.
>
> —Hegel, *The Phenomenology of the Spirit*

Everything I have said so far points in the direction of the supreme importance of mourning in the human unconscious. For, on the one hand, Freud and Lacan ground the symbolic organization of the unconscious on a regime of failed mourning that goes on and on and that is based on processes of guilt, anger, shame, and the identification with the dead father. And, on the other hand, Lacan shows how the imaginary organization of the unconscious is partly based on a fear of the mother's nonpresence and the subject's own possible death. A state of mourning, then, or something closely related to it, a state of lack that has to be mourned, lies at the heart of the formation of the unconscious for both men; a state of mourning that is tied to the subject's isolation or absence from the other, of being alone, but also that is tied to the horror of having committed an unspeakable offense against the Other, as in the sense of when the brother cries: "What have I done, where is my father?" and in the sense of when the infant cries for its absent mother whom it has made disappear in its fantasies, as happens, for instance, when a child throws a spool across the screen of a baby's crib. And, while the Lacanian Imaginary subject may answer his cry by saying that "I am whole and complete in myself," and while Freud's brother may respond that he has become his own father by identifying the desire of the father with his own desire, both responses to loss are triggered by narcissistic reactions, the consequence of which is that the subject cannot recall the lost object except as an ideal or as an Imaginary mirror image of the Other's desire.

But, we may stop and wonder, what is really being mourned in the unconscious? Is it the fact that the subject must face the future alone and that he feels vulnerable in his loneliness? Does the absence of the mother or the father recall the dependency of infancy, or the easy loss of life—easy come, easy go? Or is it something else? Is the thing that is being ambivalently mourned not a person or a state (like absence) at all? Perhaps mourning is a way to remember the dead without acknowledging a desire that the other disappears, or that the subject itself is gone. Mourning would then be a symptom of an impulse to prohibit a wish that the subject enjoys the drive to make disappear and to destroy, that is, that the subject ambivalently enjoys the death drive.

What does it mean to say that the unconscious mourns instead of acknowledging the subject's enjoyment in making itself, or some other person or object, disappear or, in acknowledging the subject's enjoyment in breaking things up, in smashing them, and in seeing them fall apart? Freud provides only limited, and somewhat enigmatic, help when he writes his strange genealogy of the unconscious's relation to death in "On War" (1915). Nevertheless, it is to it that I want to turn for help in explaining these issues. To begin with, elsewhere, Freud insists that the unconscious has no way to represent negation to itself, hence it can have no understanding of death or even of the idea of "No." But in "On War" (1915), he writes, not for the first or the last time, that people at first tried to keep death at a distance, that is, to not acknowledge that they can die. They did not want to accept the idea that life is structured by dying and so they kept it from entering consciousness. They took no notice, or, rather, they made nothing much out of it, only enjoying killing strangers, without attaching any signs of horror or grief to the deed. But, to kill a stranger did not make them ponder the inevitability of their own death. These early humans only "tasted . . . grief" when they saw someone whom they loved, and who they felt was a part of themselves, die. It was when these dear others died that they felt the first pangs of mortality and grief so that, as Freud writes, the shadow of the object fell over their ego.

Now, listen to what Freud says next, because it contains a genealogy of the subject's unconscious relation to mourning as much as a genealogy of the subject's unconscious relation to death; or, rather, it ties the two together. Even when he felt the bitterness of loss, when he grieved, this early human "still could not consent entirely to acknowledge it, for he could not conceive of himself as dead." This is curious, unless Freud means that this first grieving man faced internal resistance to extending the possibility of dying to himself. He could not conceive the possibility that he would really die.

We can distinguish at least two sources of this resistance. The first form of resistance is contained in the wish to deny something unpleasant, and this source of resistance is undoubtedly the main resistance Freud had in mind in 1915 since it is prima facie the work of the pleasure principle. But, there is a second form of resistance behind this wish to deny something unpleasant; but, it is a source that only becomes self-evident to Freud after he formulates the death drive: it is the wish to deny the enjoyment in facing what Freud will call the death drive; that is, these early humans felt a resistance to acknowledge the selfsame drive to self-disunion, self-disappearance, and death that Freud sees as the repressed thing lurking behind the installation of the superego in the unconscious and in the unconscious compulsion to mourn the loss of the father through guilt, through inhibitions, through anxieties, and through symptoms. Here, all that he says, however, is that this individual had to overcome some internal resistance to the idea of his own death, that is, to his own final disappearance. So, Freud concludes here that "he devised a compromise: he conceded the fact of death, even his own death, but denied it the significance of annihilation, which he had no motive of contesting where the death of his enemy had been concerned." From this compromise, wrote Freud, came the entire animistic world and the world of ghosts. That the motivation behind the creation of a ghostly world for the dead-but-not-completely-gone was a compromise based in a need to mourn is revealed in the following sentence, when Freud adds: "During the contemplation of his loved one's corpse he invented ghosts, and it was his sense of guilt at the satisfaction mingled with his sorrow that turned these new-born spirits into evil, dreaded demons."[1] Thus, he invented evil spirits so that he can go on mourning free of those hostile impulses to take pleasure in the disappearance of the deceased—that is, not to take pleasure in what Freud will call, five years on, the subject's turning its death drive against the Other. The lesson to be drawn from this brief genealogy of death and mourning, then, is that this kind of mourning in the unconscious has the structural purpose of acknowledging death but not the death drive, of allowing the loss and the love for those whom we love and who are gone, but not the enjoyment the subject takes in their being gone, entering consciousness.

In *The Interpretation of Dreams* (1900) Freud already described how the subject can enjoy the death of someone while keeping that enjoyment out of consciousness, but he does so without fully knowing what he is saying. In other words, the admixture of the pleasure taken in the death of the person one loves had to be partly repressed by the subject's conscious grief for the deceased person so the subject can mourn, but the persistence of these negative feelings in the unconscious also became the cause of the persistence of evil spirits, of the inability to let the dead rest, and of the constant haunting of the living by the dead. And, it is just the smallest step to take, one I believe Freud makes after he formulates the dual drive theory, to say that the reason the subject unconsciously mourns in this way stems from the fact that the subject cannot acknowledge the enjoyment it takes in destruction of the other, and in the subject's own wish to disunion, disintegration, falling apart, and to destroy itself.

Rather than mourn the dead and then turn our libido elsewhere, the unconscious subject is haunted by its own past and by the return of its hostile wishes as ghosts, Freud writes, even if these ghosts do not always appear in the "standard edition."[2] These ghosts, however, do appear behind our guilt, our slips of the tongue, our slips of the pen, and our symptoms.[3] That is to say, the subject creates a whole world of ghosts and specters to avoid facing what Freud calls, after 1920, the ambivalent desire to take pleasure in disunion and in destroying ourselves and the other as a proxy of ourselves. In the same way, the subject in our unconscious mourns and mourns, and it creates one ghostly apparition after another because the unconscious has become structured to maintain the prohibition against the enjoyment of the disappearances and deaths of those we loved in this way.

The subject, thus, acknowledges death as a source of grief and loss, as Freud says, but does so by not acknowledging something else: the enjoyment the subject takes in the death drive and the wish that the subject, or the other, disappear. It should be clear by now that this impulse not only stems from the drives that are located in our body, but that it also originates in our well-defended narcissism. At other times, Freud says that we poor humans are forced, by reason of our premature birth, to flee reality into a world of narcissistic illusions so that we can maintain the prohibition residing in our unconscious.[4] At first, he limits the prohibited thing to incest. And, originally, the installation of the father-complex is only accompanied by the incest taboo (guarded by guilt and castration anxiety). But, the dual drive theory calls for a revision to this theory of the prohibited thing—even if Freud never explicitly makes the revision himself. Now, we can see that the unconscious compulsion to mourn the death of the father requires the *jouissance* of the death drive also be prohibited. This is, after all, just what the society of brothers do according to Freud, and what, also according to Freud, each one of us continues to do ourselves: We and they collectively forget the murder which must have included the enjoyment of destroying the father. Instead, we and they misremember the pleasure we took for an instant in being in the place of the primal father. Instead of giving in to the pleasure again, we and they install a repeating, unending, guilty compulsion to mourn a repressed loss and an ambivalent love of the father—a father whom the subject loves so much that it both installs a Symbolic father at the center of its psyche, at the point of its most intimate identifications, and that it, thereby, mourns unconsciously, but does so, at least in part in order to not recall the enjoyment it once felt in doing the deed, and in the disappearance of the Other. Thus, the subject's enjoyment in the exercise of the death drive is replaced by an act of mourning, or perhaps the subject's *jouissance* in the death drive gets replaced by an act of monumentalizing. In fact, the connection to monuments goes farther since, as in the case of erecting a war monument, it is a question of the subject monumentalizing loss, but not the *jouissance* of the death drive; that is, while the subject grieves disappearance, it forgets the *jouissance* it once took in the act of desiring or causing the other to disappear. Something like what occurs, for example, when Freud's patient wished that her sister would die so that her sister's husband would become free to marry her. But, like them, we misremember the substitution of this pleasure with an ambivalent identification with the Law.

Once this becomes a component of our unconscious (to varying degrees), the subject is caught up in a compulsive act of remembering and forgetting, of endless mourning. We are pushed hither and thither by love and guilt, but we are pushed and pulled in this fashion so that the subject does not respond to another desire: a desire to enjoy disunion, disintegration, disappearance, and death.

Even in 1915, five years before he publishes his dual drive theory, Freud is explicit on this point. By refusing to acknowledge the enjoyment of death, by making it disappear into a spirit world where the dead live on, a spirit world from which comes evil punishing spirits, the subject takes the first steps toward religion, civilization, and morality. That is, the subject takes the first steps into a world in which the *jouissance* of this death drive will be circumscribed by more and more prohibitions and where guilt and remorse become the tools of symbolic repression of the subject and its desires. The creation of ghosts and evil spirits are, then: "the earliest inkling of ethical law." The commandment Thou Shall Not Kill marks the grave stone over a repressed injunction against remembering the subject's experience of his death drive.

We have a whole genealogy here, once we read the prohibition of the death drive into the prohibition to kill, which goes as follows: Religion, ethics, and civilization develop from the prohibition to kill, a prohibition that itself springs from the subject's guilt and fear of the dead, but this fear is already a construct of other fears that rest in the prohibition of the subject to enjoy the death drive. The generation by humans of a spirit world, and the forms of mourning it allows them, therefore, are psychic scenes to keep the subject from acknowledging the pleasure it takes in causing something to disappear or die. One terminus place where this sort of mourning leads can be found in Georges Bataille's description of the social and psychological phenomena of the potlatch (where American Indian Eskimo chiefs vied with each other over who can destroy their wealth in great festivals of waste and excess), or in Bataille's discussion of Aztec human sacrifice (which occurred in huge dramatic social festivals of excess as well). In these extravagant social and symbolic acts, the satisfaction-in-destroying is just barely masked by the respectable veneer of instrumental goals including putting the chief's wealth and power on display (the potlatch) and appeasing the gods to assure the New Year's harvest (Aztec human sacrifice).[5] These societies, then, maintain the social bond through mediated and symbolic acts of violence that reveal the communal pleasure in destruction but then they rationalize these acts as being something else, just as the individual rationalizes his or her conduct by finding other reasons to justify his or her violent behavior. Or, rather, we see here that the thing that is being prohibited from becoming conscious is not the enjoyment in destruction per se, which is what I have been saying, but rather the thing that is being prohibited is for the subject to acknowledge that this lust for destruction on which the social bond rests can not be justified—except to rationalize the extent to which the subject finds satisfaction in these acts of disunity, disintegrating, making things come undone, and finally ceasing to be. This process of hiding the prohibition of a *jouissance* in destruction behind a rationalization has, if anything, become far more common in modern society. But, Freud suggests, it is a human dilemma and not just a product of modernization that the subject erects rituals and ethical injunctions against acknowledging its enjoyment in destruction.

The resistance to acknowledging a piece of reality, for Freud, is the problem. If people truly transcended the enjoyment that they take in violence and in things falling apart, if they really were ethical creatures, everything would be fine. They would mourn loss and then move on to new loves, but, in fact, at least at the level of the unconscious, this is not how the subject mourns. Rather, the subject mourns in order to maintain the prohibition, and behind the prohibition lurks the subject's continuing pleasure in the death drive. Hence, it is the unconscious relation between the pleasure in destroying and in the enactment of the prohibition of acknowledging this pleasure (which has its own pleasure, too) which the subject cannot rise above. We have, therefore, by mourning in this way, only begun to figure out as a partly conscious life form how to live ethically given the existence of this pleasure in destruction. But it is a beginning that keeps the subject circling round and round the site of a massacre without ever getting anywhere else. This is the essence of trauma for Freud: the compulsion to repeat, the need to constantly return to the moment of catastrophe, because one cannot free one's libido from it.

If, phylogenetically speaking, mourning covers over the loss of the father, Melanie Klein, who develops Freud's work into the dangerous world of the death drive and Eros, but without showing even the slightest interest in his phylogenetic arguments, has a different but not unrelated position on the question of the unacknowledged pleasure we take in destruction. For Klein, enjoyment in destruction is something that appears repeatedly in the subject's fantasies about the mother or about parts of the mother's body. Specifically, the Kleinian baby is a needy, loving, but also murderous child, which is why for Klein the whole point of psychic development is for the child to move from a paranoid-schizoid position where life remains fragmented, split, and constantly in danger of falling apart to a depressive and then a post-depressive position where the child's world is composed of whole objects and where the desire to destroy, tear apart, poison, and steal, which remain impulses even in the depressive and post-depressive position, are effectively opposed by impulses to repair, tolerance, and gratitude for the other.

With Klein, we begin to see the turn from triangles based on the child-mother-father relation to mother-child relationship. Hence, for Klein, the first experiential loss in the life of a child involves the infant's mother (or the part object associated to what the child will later recognize to be a part of the mother), and, therefore, the mother is the first and most important object that the subject fears losing or destroying. And, while the object-relations turn away from drives will be pursued by Fairbairn, Southerland, and others in a much more radical way than Klein, it was she who defined many of the most original and radical concepts developed in object relations theory, including projective identification and envy. To begin with, in general Klein stressed that projective mechanisms push the death drive outside the self part of the mind by, in essence, denying death a home within the self part of the ego. That is, it makes the effects of the death drive *unheimlich*, thereby reinforcing the emerging difference between an experience of a "me" world and a (usually bad) "not me" world. Klein, therefore, shows how the death drive is from the very beginning of the life of the infant already disavowed and denied a home in its emerging experience of a "me" world, except as paranoid assaults from the "not-me" world associated with external object and with the internal world of bad objects. One can see that splitting, which is also designed to deny the death drive a place in the "me" world, paradoxically works to increase, rather than decrease, the child's flight from reality into what Klein calls fantasy.[6] For example, a child may defend itself against paranoid attacks from the object by generating defensive manic fantasies that are grandiose and over-idealized and which distort the infant's perception of so-called external reality, too.

Another way the ego tries to project its hostile feelings onto bad objects is through the very primitive defense of projective identification. The projective-identifier, according to Klein, displaces his usually hostile emotions into the mind of another person, a mental action that allows the subject to form an identification with these feelings that are now located in the other as if they are emotionally a part of the subject that it has rediscovered in the other. Hence, projective identification allows the building up of a complex interpersonal object relations world when the self and object still remain deeply confused and intermingled in the child's mind. It turns the other into an emotional puppet who feels the negative and less commonly positive emotions of the subject for it. Thus, projective identification is ideal for the displacement of feelings of inner envy for the good object onto an external object (which is still felt by the child to be partly part of the self) from where it can be reintrojected into the self as if it originated in another person.

Projective identification, being a very primitive defense, often is associated by Klein with feelings of rage, fragmentation, chaos, and the ego's falling to bits. Yet, the impulse to destroy, tear, and poison the object, or the self, parts of the mind reaches its zenith in the Kleinian concept of envy. Klein defines envy in two ways. In one: "Envy is the angry feeling that another person possesses and enjoys something desirable—the envious impulse being to take it away or to spoil it."[7] The other definition, which by all standards is more basic, defines envy as a very primal and pure manifestation of what Freud in another context calls a culture of the death drive. Here, what is at issue is not despoiling something good that the other possesses but in destroying goodness itself; and, since envy originates in oral-sadistic and anal-sadistic impulses, the envious person takes pleasure in destroying the good breast and its imaginary contents first.

Klein held the view that envy is a pervasive expression of the death drive in which love is almost completely absent; and, she asserts that "frustration and unhappy circumstances rouse some envy and hate throughout life"[8] when it is not restrained by counter-feelings of gratitude, love, and regret; bearing in mind that gratitude, too, can become a form of resisting reality, rather than acknowledging it when the subject over-idealizes the object. Thus, even after the psyche has developed well beyond the depressive position, there are always points of tension that occur which will threaten the integration of the ego with disunion, disintegration, and regression because an envious person "cannot stop . . . but must pursue the satisfaction to its logical end and destroy what it desires leaving the ego subject to paranoid and sadistic attacks."[9]

The death drive is at its zenith, in the Kleinian baby, at or near birth, when the mental structures that inhibit the death drives are unformed and when, consequently, Eros appears weakest. This may also be the moment when envy is at its peak, too, since Klein believes that the baby is object-seeking at birth, and envy defines the baby taking oral-sadistic and anal-sadistic satisfaction in destroying the good life-affirming object. If the reader wants a clinical application of envy, consider the alcoholic who cannot restrain his oral need for drink; instead, he disregards the inhibition, which he accepts in other areas of his life, and he pays by being subjected to the severe judgments of his superego and also with a regression to an oral-sadistic pleasure in destroying what is good and life-affirming about himself to such an extent that he denies his drinking problem until it is almost too late.[10] As we already saw, envy is also connected with a fragmentation of the ego and it is for this reason that envy so often can be equated with the subject feeling as if it is falling into bits—that is, with schizoid mechanisms.

For Freud as well, and this is one of the meanings of the primal murder mythology for him, the subject is already born into a world in which its death drive is prematurely developed and its life drive is prematurely weak. That is, the subject is born into a world where, phylogenetically speaking, the unconscious is already structured around the absence of the father, except in the displaced form of the superego because the deed has already occurred (the Symbolic order is already in place), and, as Lacan will add later on, because the deed has occurred already there is a need on the part of the subject to prohibit the *jouissance* of the death drive from entering into consciousness. That is, the subject is born into a certain mourning-form. The child's entry into the Symbolic order will depend on the fact that these forms of mourning and forgetting are directed along certain proscribed historical pathways.[11]

This makes people doubly alienated. On the one hand, they feel alienated by the loss of some *jouissance* that is being held under prohibition, when the subject cannot gain access to a piece of reality as part of the price of entering the Symbolic order (of gaining access to language).[12] However, another form of alienation emerges from the fact that the subject cannot acknowledge the pleasure it takes in disappearing and death. At least it cannot acknowledge this pleasure without running afoul of the superego; that is, it cannot acknowledge to itself that the forms of pleasures that it gains access to are forever lacking something and being sustained by something that they cannot gain any proper access to.

Any signification is lacking and cannot have direct access to the primal Thing. Instead, our knowledge always remains incomplete and, therefore, partly in error because all thought is already under the sign of a primal cut and castration. By speaking of alienation and the subject in this way, we are also speaking about the paradoxical space of presence and absence where (when it says something) the subject is nevertheless constantly speaking about nothing—that is, it is speaking *sotto* voce to itself about the Thing that it cannot have access to in the world opened up to it by linguistic forms of desire. Yet, we cannot stop speaking about what we cannot know or what we can only know through the signs and symptoms left by its absence.

This constant mourning also refers to the register of the Real for Lacan and it also is the Thing that Freud finds in the navel of the dream—an ultimate nothingness beyond representation and desire. A state of lack and tension that is connected to an experience of being cut off from the source of a pleasure that can only exist in Nature and which can only make its appearance in the realm of desire and representation by being coupled with guilt and repression; that is, it can only appear coupled to a sign.

In fact, Freud describes negation exactly along these lines. Negation is that which only appears in the unconscious through the hole or absence it leaves. For Freud, the positive indication of negation always misses its mark: "You may think I am referring to my mother, but I assure you doctor. . . ." or else it appears as a sign of a hole in consciousness. One can think of castration anxiety (the hole that desire seeks to fill in) as the quintessential sign of the negative. This at any rate is precisely what Freud does in works like *Inhibition, Symptom, and Anxiety* (1927). And, in this way, by linking the negative to the positive signs of castration, he suggests we think about negativity as the other side of desire and representation, as the underbelly of the images and words in the unconscious.

To review what we have concluded thus far in this chapter: negation (under repression) lies at the base of the unconscious, and the subject can have access to some pleasures, but not to others. Apropos this, the first form of negation Freud discusses was the "No" associated to incest. Later, he will broaden the realm of the negative by advancing the idea of a death drive (André Green has been especially good at examining this world of the negative in recent years).

Pleasures, such as are available hereafter, are shallowed-out pleasures, the pleasures we know being displaced from some other pleasure that the subject can only know through the symptom: a substitute-pleasure connected with another negated and prohibited pleasure that we do not know. And, from this vantage, the defenses are structured at least in part to restrain the pleasure in the destruction of the self or the Other and in incest prohibited by the Law.

Apropos this, Freud discusses at least three forms of restraint that allow individuals to live with themselves and others. There is the restraint of the primal father's society: a restraint based on a mixture of love and fear of being punished and, ultimately, killed. Lest one thinks that this form of restraint has been superseded, Freud states in many places ranging from "On War" (1915) to *Civilization and Its Discontents* (1930) that most people are only superficially ethical and that they therefore restrain their narcissism out of fear of punishment more than out of an identification with the Right (whatever Kant believed). There also is a form of restraint that emerges, Freud writes, following the resolution of the oedipal complex: a restraint that is more internal than external and which, Freud argues, is associated with the installation of the superego in the psyche and which draws the mind into varieties of neurotic symptoms, and whose form is self-restraint out of a fear of self-castration which we can describe as the Symbolic substitution for murder à la Oedipal act of self-blinding. Finally, there is the self-restraint that Freud only implies in some of his writings. I will call this the self-restraint of an ideal-Moses.[13] The character of the ideal-Moses is such that a large piece of the reality that has to be repressed by the superego and substituted by symptoms and anxiety will no longer be kept from our field of perception. As a result, where the whole point of oedipal structure was to sustain a certain mourning-form at the base of morality and civilization, the new form of restraint would allow more of the formerly prohibited enjoyment access to consciousness. In other words, more of the prohibited *jouissance* would be tolerated without triggering a need to compulsively cover over the satisfaction and replace it with guilt and remorse.

What I have been saying is intended to highlight the hope that less symptomatic forms of mourning are not only possible but that these new forms of mourning mean we need not continue to repeat the same old established mourning structures simply because it is being kept under prohibition or is being opposed by powerful feelings of guilt and anxiety. This comment, however, requires its own further clarification: what I have just said about developing a new relation to the need to mourn does not mean that the current subject cannot represent and feel enjoyment in destruction—for this is something he or she obviously does—it is the very basis of his or her unconscious Imaginary and Symbolic sadistic and masochistic symptoms and signifiers. Of course, the subject does come to know, or can be made through introspection to know, pleasure in destruction and disharmony. But this way of knowing one's desires remains overly ambivalent, based as it is on an unacknowledged tension between the prohibited Thing, the unconscious world of representations, and the unique history of each and every one of us.

The reader may be wondering at this moment: what sorts of knowledge can this produce for the subject? Certainly, it is not comforting in the sense that we speak of when we comfort the sick and mourning soul by filling their heads with pleasantries and consolations. Neither is it the sort of knowledge that seeks to teach people how to substitute the pain of loss with what Martin Heidegger and Alexandre Kojevé called the flight into distraction. Nor is it something akin to the art of escaping from the Real into an ideal world of Beauty or Truth. Above all, it is emphatically not a withdrawal from the Real into the world of narcissism and pleasure-seeking. Rather, it is the sort of knowledge that helps the subject bear, but not idealize, its separation in the Real; and, on the level of object relations, it is the kind of knowledge that allows the subject to develop new desires—ones less beholden to a compulsion to mourn in the old ways.

Lacan suggests a way to conceptualize this break with the old forms of desire and restraint when he says that people need to acquire a new *savoir-faire*, a new way of knowing that is simultaneously connected to his analysis of the four discourses, which I will get to momentarily, and to this problematic and enigmatic project, that is already there in an unfinished form in Freud's text *Beyond the Pleasure Principle* (1920), that we psychoanalysts become the birth-mothers of a new development in the history of the spirit.

Thus, in his schema of the four discourses, Lacan equates the discourse of the unconscious with the Master's discourse, which he writes in the following manner:

$$\frac{S_1}{\$} \quad \frac{S_2}{a} \quad \text{(Master's discourse)}$$

The Master discourse that Lacan has in mind here is related to the logic of the subject who submits to the desire of the Other by treating the analyst as the "person supposed to know," that is, the person who can fill the analysand in on what he or she must do and how he or she must be. The subject who submits to this form of unconscious discourse accepts his or her dependence on the desire of the Other and we can say that he or she remains locked in a discourse where the subject, like a child, defines itself by realizing the desire of the Other.

But what the Master is supposed to know, or what the Master is supposed to desire, cannot fill in the subject's unconscious sense of lack, nor can it cover over the gap that exists between the repressed *jouissance* and the world of signifiers in the unconscious. This discourse, then, is built on a series of self-deceits and duplicities. The Master supposed to know actually covers over the fact that the Master is not the holder of any truth about the subject's missing *jouissance*. By the same token, the one who is seduced by the Master's discourse, the person who makes the Master out to be the one supposed to know remains subject to never knowing his own desire but to only realizing himself by realizing the Other's desire. The discourse of the Master, therefore, is really a discourse that sustains a logic of domination based on an illusion.[14]

Alternatively, Lacan represents the Analyst's discourse in this way:

$$\frac{a}{S_1} \quad \frac{\$}{S_2} \quad \text{(Analyst's discourse)}$$

The Analyst's discourse, in other words, turns the logic of the Master's discourse on its side. Here, the analysand moves a good deal in the direction of what Freud asks for when he says that people need to acknowledge death's role in our psyches a little more because now the analyst only claims to know, to speak, the truth of the object a; that is to say, the analyst is not the spokesperson of the Symbolic. To become the spokesperson of the Symbolic is what Lacan thought the ego psychologist aspired to be. Nor is the psychoanalyst a spokesperson of the Imaginary as many of the new schools of psychoanalysis focusing on the mother-child relation to the exclusion of the Symbolic and the Real aspire to be. Rather, if one can speak this way at all, Lacan makes the analyst into a cipher who stands in for the non-present Real, and calls to the analysand to speak the truth of his own desire (that is of his symptom). This project, I may add, is something that is reminiscent of the Sphinx who asked Oedipus the question which allowed the Theban prince to speak his own desire not once but three times, since Oedipus speaks it again at the end of "Oedipus Rex" and then again in "Oedipus at Colona."

Another way of getting at the relationship between the subject and the Other implicit in this Analyst discourse is to take note of the structural role that negation and lack perform in it; because, unlike the Master's discourse, in the Analyst's discourse the analysand's desire does not rest in the illusion that he or she can come to hold the truth that the analyst knows but is not revealing to them. Similarly, the analysand is barred from attempting to realize his or her own desire by the path of satisfying the desire of the Other. And, surely, we are only stretching things a little if we add that abjuring the desire of the Other as one's own desire must include abjuring the logic of unconscious mourning that leads to the identification with the dead father I developed before, whereas this is just what the brothers do in Freud's great myth of the birth of the Symbolic order when the brothers as a community identify their desire with the Law. Instead, the subject must find his own desire in the slow work of the analysis of the letters, words, and signifiers of his own unconscious.

This allows for a very different sort of relation between the analysand and the analyst where the analyst functions less as the one supposed to know. As a consequence, a different sort of adventure can begin for the analysand. Alain-Miller more or less says this when he notes that "Lacan formulates the possibility of psychoanalysis as the distance between big I (S1) for little a."[15] Or, when he adds, later in the same talk, that "the fall of the subject supposed to know implies the replacement of this signification by object a."[16] But one has to mention that beyond allowing the analysand to discover his or her own desire rather than to fix one's sights on satisfying the desire of the other, what this encounter with the representation of the Real (the object a) amounts to remains clouded in controversy. Some Lacanians are drawn by it into a sort of mysticism of a *jouissance* beyond the object; some others are attracted to a sense of a *jouissance* and a logic of desire spun out without the safety-net of the Master's Truth in the background. Others are drawn to a Levinasian ethic of openness to the other free of any controlling Law mediating how the two shall be with each other.

Because I am not qualified to judge between them, I will simply return to Freud and mention that he, too, was interested in bringing the unconscious desires of the patients to a new place that would be beyond the place where our desires had to be founded in the desire of a God-father complex. In other words, rather than sustain the subject in the Symbolic order, Freud wants desire to be founded only in itself and in the world of Nature which it is partly a part of. And, apropos this, overcoming the unconscious compulsion to mourn in the old ways should therefore be seen as a piece of this larger project, carried forward by Lacan, of finding a new grounding for desire in a demystified world (read as a world not ordered around the old logic of the Symbolic order). The way forward that was taken in the past, Freud suggests, began a process of interminable mourning so that the subject would not acknowledge its murderous yearning to disappear by binding lack to the wheel of guilt and castration anxiety. But continuing down this path leads literally nowhere—except the endless repetition and disavowal of trauma. Perhaps, if we could acknowledge our real attachments to the pleasure in disappearing and in making others disappear, we could find a more realistic and less destructive way forward at last.

Finding a new way forward that is ground in a more realistic appraisal of *jouissance* and desire also raises the question of nomination that I mentioned before. For, in the past, in Europe's medieval and early modern periods, kings claimed to be nominated by God. This Symbolic nomination implied a whole make-believe relation between the king, the body politic, and God who guaranteed the king's position in society. This does not mean that this form of the Master's discourse was ever the only one in play. In fact, this discourse was always contested by other discourses in medieval, early modern, and modern European societies. For example, later, through Rousseau, this nomination passed to the people, but without changing the fundamental logic of the nomination, which still remained bogged in the repetition of the old forms of mourning.

If we read this process of Symbolic legitimation from a Freudian angle then we can say that gaining this sort of legitimacy gave to its holder some of the power that a perpetual unconscious state of mourning grants to the name of the father, whereas psychoanalysis seeks a radically different relation between desire and the Other. Perhaps Freud suggests what that different relation may look like when he tells us in "Mourning and Melancholia" (1917) that the ego can kill itself only when it treats itself "as an object." This would help explain how the death drive and the pleasures in destruction goes about overwhelming the drive to life and union; and it therefore may also point a way to a desiring subject who no longer is stuck in the compulsion to constantly replace the death drive with the signs of guilt that turn the subject or the other into an object of moral reproach and punishment. If we could do that a radically new relation between the subject and the other may arise not based on trying to manipulate or appease the desire of the other. Perhaps, then, Levinas is the true successor to this part of Freud's legacy.

I will not say much more about this here because much still remains undecidable, but this much I can say, at least. If by facing the enjoyment the subject takes in disappearing (as well as in appearing) the subject finds the lever to overcome its interminable need to mourn in the same old ways by symbolically returning to the scene of the crime again and again, then we still may find new and better ways of being with others in spite of our ongoing ambivalent attraction to disharmony, destruction, and disunion. At the very least, by overcoming the compulsion to mourn in the same old way in order not to feel the absence of a kind of *jouissance*, the subject will be able to remove one of the most pernicious obstacles separating it from the other; and, as a result, it may discover its bonds to the past and the future generations (the unions of Eros) are more secure and well-grounded than it imagined. It is not that the ambivalence of love and hate will disappear, but what may change is how the subject experiences these conflicting impulses. Something new may yet appear that may help the subject to overcome a certain impasse to desire brought on by the unconscious compulsion to repeat an old form of mourning. And, in this way, by bringing these two domains of subject-other and of drive-representation nearer to one another, the subject may lessen the degree of psychic tension and the power of the symptom that it has to bear, because the weight of its discontents will be less.

Ultimately, this new knowledge should allow the subject to free more libido so that it can go out and find new objects, and so lessen its discontentment and alienation and this will have the beneficial consequence of helping the subject get over its angers and disunions with those whom it loves and whose loss it may already be mourning, like Freud's two companions who were lost in anticipatory mourning. And, as a result, the subject will be able to sustain its ties to others in spite of the influence of the death drive and, rather than escaping into a world of narcissism and distraction, the subject will be more inclined to feel its connection to those who came before and are now gone, those whom the subject loves who are still here, and those future generations whom it will never know; that is, it will be able to accept its place in the chain of life.

To have a legacy is to be bound to the past and the future, to find one's place in the chain of generations. To be able to take one's place in the generation of generations not only fixes us in time but it also places us with the Other (rather than in some Imaginary or Symbolic space where we are somehow unique, complete, and an exception to the normal order of things): Not the Imaginary man in the mirror or the signifier of phallic authority, but someone. On the drive level, this new knowledge reinforces the work of Eros uniting with others to form greater wholes to further the work of civilization and to also further the work of the moral development of the individual. But what it is not is a regression to an Imaginary state of Oneness where the narcissistic ego feels grandiose. Nor is it a return to an imagined merger (such as Freud warns against in many of his writings) where the ego is swallowed whole by the other. One is tied to the other without swallowing it up or being swallowed up by it. One has a place but it is not the place of the king any more.

It is only this later sort of knowledge that will be capable of sustaining a subject who is able to find his or her way to their own desire, the operative assumption being that finding one's own desire may be tied to finding a different relation to mourning and the death drive. If one likes, one can say that this knowledge sustains the sort of subject who resembles King Oedipus no more than he or she resembles King Lear. Instead this is a subject who like Hamlet pretends madness and like that fool of twentieth-century cinema, Charlie Chaplin, knows how to fall and then pick himself up without too much fuss. And, apropos this, the subject learns to become a performer, a "tightrope walker" as Nietzsche may say, and an expert in the pratfall, the stumble, and the flip. That is, an expert in the slip up without the complete breakdown or without completely losing one's footing.

In conclusion, I have argued that mourning has played an important structural role in the formation of the unconscious. In one sense, mourning is like a dam that the subject erects against the torrents of the drives and that the subject subsequently covers up by other defenses. These metaphors for mourning—a bridge, a dam, a screen—however, fail to do justice to the primacy of mourning in the structure of the unconscious and the relation between the subject and the other that is under discussion. For what Freud's entire oeuvres strongly implies is the idea that the need to mourn pathologically lies at the origin of our morality, our civilization, and our individual developments and fixations. It shapes the very ways we desire and establish relations to the other.

Let me, therefore, try to approach this from a different angle by way of bringing this chapter to a close. In the formation of the unconscious, and in the relations between the unconscious subject and the Other, mourning plays a pivotal role in the defenses. And, if we pursue this, we will see that mourning is also the scene of a trauma and a repetition compulsion pushed under the bar of repression by the other defenses. We have a situation, then, where the actions of the drives which are pre-representational are represented for the unconscious as a scene of traumatic mourning in which the subject's desire is constantly running afoul of feelings of coming undone or when the subject is constantly running afoul of manic defenses against the unconscious representation of death.

Given this situation which forms the Symbolic universe into which every generation is born, it is the aim of psychoanalysis, in my opinion, to eventually push back the rock to reveal the subject's own unique desire to him or her self covered over by the need to mourn. This will lessen not only the compulsion to repeat an old act of mourning, it also will fundamentally alter the subject's relation to its own drives. In fact, the place of death, and the place of the death drive, will undergo a fundamental change so that the subject will be more able to promote, rather than inhibit, the work of its own Eros toward union and the elaboration of life. The subject's relation to herself and to the other will also change such that the subject will no longer be as preoccupied with the Eros that falls apart; and, instead, the subject will become more able to turn its freed libido toward expanding and deepening its erotic ties to others. And, whereas the old forms of mourning produced reserves of guilt, the new forms of mourning will produce something different. And, whereas the old forms of mourning lead the subject to a compulsion to use guilt to inhibit desire—especially the desire to do "bad things"—and to keep watch on oneself so that one does not blame the real source of one's ambivalence, the new form of mourning will place the subject in a completely different relation to their guilt.

Apropos guilt and the subject, feelings of guilt and remorse will be especially powerful for people who have suffered a premature exposure to their death drives, who are predisposed to a higher than normal quantity of death drives, or who have been victims of traumas and health problems in their life. For people suffering from these sorts of weaknesses or regressions, the best hope is that when they are overwhelmed by persecutory (and other early forms of excessive) death drives the boundary can be maintained and the resident eventually brought within a Symbolic order. But once they have made this transition we must help the subject who has learned to transpose her death wishes into guilt and remorse to recover the lack sustaining the guilt. For the analytic cure by these lights will be based in part on how successful the analyst is in helping the analysand modify the structure of his or her unconscious, at the point where the drives to union and disunion are transferred onto a representational field or words, letters, narratives, affects, and defenses. For, everything I have said so far suggests that the representational level of the unconscious will tend to be stuck in a compulsion repeating a trauma about the death of the subject. Sometimes, these images of death will be transformed into a representation of the persecution by bad objects, or they will be transformed into the unconscious obsession with representations about the death of the other. At other times, these death images will be transformed into affects like guilt, remorse, and the punishment of the subject's desires, although we are no nearer to explaining how this transition occurs today than in Freud's day.

This is far from a consoling way to end this chapter, but we can say one thing that may soften its edge a little: if we fail to see our way into the future, it will be largely because we have failed to overcome our past trauma enough to get beyond a compulsion to mourn. But the great collective experiment of civilization may yet come out well if we can find better means to express our prohibited forms of *jouissance*. That is, perhaps our future survival may hinge on what we do with our death drives other than try to repress or convert them into moral commandments. But perhaps, if we give death its place in our psychic economy, as Freud suggests, the subject can move beyond the cycles of mourning, guilt, remembrance, and repression to a new ethics based on a greater knowledge of who we are and what our possibilities are.[17]

This is a strange journey we are on. Beginning from the need to lift the prohibition against the enjoyment in disunion and disharmony a little, we have arrived back to the question of what is possible. Is this simply shirking the hard work of facing the death drive? Perhaps. But I cannot help believe that the lessening of the prohibition will have more positive than negative consequences and that it, ultimately, will reduce the discontent the subject feels in civilization. That is, it also will lessen the flight into neurosis and psychosis. And, that can only be a good thing.

Perhaps we can tie this hope to Freud's suggestion that by completing the process of mourning, the subject can free its libido to go out and find new objects—thus expanding the universe of Eros again. A choice, therefore, exists between whether we will remain fixated in our old compulsions to mourn in a certain fashion or struggle to make them conscious.

This brings the first part of this book to its conclusion. The second half of this book develops my experience as an analyst and psychologist working with men and women in a number of nursing homes. As a result, it will concern itself with people facing death, preoccupied with their mortality or the mortality of others, and sometimes, very rarely, with their place in the chain of life. Some residents in the nursing home will express their fears and obsession in largely oedipal forms, many others will address their anxieties from pre-oedipal positions. And we will see the struggle they face is our own too, since no one knows the hour of their death.

NOTES

1. Freud, "Thoughts for the Times on War and Death," 1915.
2. Freud describes how the return of the repressed distorts conscious communications through slips including those of a "Lieutenant X" who while recovering in an army hospital misreads a line of poetry as "am I alone to live? *Why should not I?*" instead of the correct lines "am I alone to live then? *Why should I?*" Sigmund Freud, *The Psychopathology of Everyday Life* in *The Complete Psychological Works of Sigmund Freud*, vol. 6 (New York: W. W. Norton & Co., 1989), 169–70.
3. A slip of the pen occurs in a bungled telegram from his publisher which reads "*Vorrate* erhalten, *Einladung* X. dringend (Provisions received, Invitation X. urgent)" instead of the correct message: "*Vorrese* erhalten, *Einleitung* X. dringend (Preface received, Introduction X. urgent)." Freud's explanation of the slip runs as follows:

> The solution of the riddle starts from the name X. mentioned in it. X. is the author of a book to which I was to write an *Einleitung* (introduction). This *Einleitung* was what had been turned into the *Einladung* (invitation). I was then able to recall that some days earlier I have sent my publisher a *Vorrese* (preface) to another book; so this was the acknowledgment of its arrival.

See Freud, *The Psychopathology of Everyday Life*, 169–70. Presumably, Freud is not the only one dreaming of provisions from abroad and, Freud concludes half-jokingly, "We may presume that it (the telegram) have fallen victim to a revision by the telegraphist's hunger-complex." And of course behind the hunger complex lay the struggle of life, orality (the mother's breast), and a deflection of the death drive.

4. Ferenczi, Freud's colleague (and Klein too) was interested in the mechanics of how more Reality is introduced into a psychic system that is at first almost completely obsessed by the need to reduce pain.

5. George Bataille, *The Accursed Share vol. 1–2*, trans. Robert Hurley (New York: Zone Books, 1991).

6. Splitting aids in the build-up of a rich object relations world by dividing the perceptions of self and object into good and bad parts that can sustain the rich Kleinian world of fantasy and defenses. Also, these same splitting mechanisms will be used to help the ego make logical distinctions later on, hence what leads to the increase in fantasy at one point leads toward a greater sense of reality later on.

7. Melanie Klein, "Envy and Gratitude," in *Envy and Gratitude* (Glencoe, Ill.: Free Press, 1984), 181.

8. Klein, "Envy and Gratitude," 190.

9. Klein, "Envy and Gratitude," 181.

10. Thus, not only is the Kleinian baby more in touch with its death drive—or at least is able to acknowledge its murderous impulses with the aide of the psychoanalyst—it also is more in touch with the enjoyment it takes in destroying even as the Kleinian baby is more "hard-wired" to master these impulses during the depressive position.

11. Apropos this, Lacan gets around Freud's seeming biologism by stating that this is a result of the fact that the unconscious is structured by words, images, letters, and linguistic narratives, and so on, that already possess a Symbolic meaning that the infant incorporates through its first interactions with its mother and father. Lacan draws a similar logic of absence or lack in his theory of desire.

12. The roots of alienation are to be found in the very nature of life so that success in transcending alienation is tantamount to returning to a tensionless state before life (Nirvana) because alienation is set in motion when life begins and disturbs the inorganic world. Marx is probably wrong to believe labor will transcend this ontological alienation between people and the world they create in part because all subjects are divided by urges to return to the inorganic state and to maintain, or increase, themselves as living systems.

13. A restraint that has nothing to do with his role as the Law-giver; it is, in fact, the antithesis of this Law-imposing Moses since one has come to more fully identify with the right without recourse to the commandments of the Other.

14. For, ultimately, what the Master is supposed to know is how to realize the analysand's desire and *jouissance* that the subject lost when the Word replaced the mute world of the drives. The trend in medicine is not toward more self-regulation, for example, but toward greater dependency on pills and on the authority of doctors who are presented to the patient as the ones who, in Lacan's phrase, are "supposed to know."

15. Miller, "Sinthome," in *Lacanian Ink 33* (New York: Wooster Press, 2009), 63.

16. Miller, "Sinthome," 66. Thus, by occupying the position of the object a, the analyst does not magically and mystically open the doors of perception to a world behind the shadows of language and desire (there is nothing there); rather, he embodies the recovery of *jouissance* (plus-de-jouir) lost when the Word covers over the drive (and replaces it with a symptom, the form of which is always to present the drives in

a weakened and diluted form so that their traumatic effects can be mastered by the symptom).

17. Play, Freud insists, not unlike Klein, uses the compulsion to repeat, to create something new not seen in the old repetition—specifically, play does not complete the circuit to the old trauma again (and Freud knew that children are exactly like adults in their attraction to repetitions and regression).

Part II

THE LONGING FOR "NOTHINGNESS" IN THE NURSING HOME

6

Introduction to Death in the Nursing Home

> What good to us is a long life if it is difficult and barren of joys, and if it is so full of misery that we can only welcome death as a deliverer?
>
> —Freud, *Civilization and Its Discontents*

The struggle between union and disunion in the depth of the unconscious is very pronounced and conscious-near in elderly people who are experiencing health problems and nearing death. One would expect that persons experiencing these sorts of problems would think about death and mortality. But it is just as common, if not more common, that, while these concerns preoccupy them unconsciously, they resist allowing these thoughts and feelings to come into consciousness. As a result, they often find themselves experiencing their concerns about mortality and death through their symptoms. They are, in other words, inclined to feel anxious or depressed or withdrawn, and when they are able, they may discuss feelings of frustration or even of things falling apart, of their lives falling into ruins; more often they may turn their anxieties and these feelings outward and blame others for causing their misfortune. They will, with rare exceptions, be able to name what is happening to them properly or to tolerate the exposure of their powerful impulses to destroy and for things to fall apart to come into consciousness without the protective shield of a projection or a symptom.

This is understandable since the amount of resistance to bringing the death drive into consciousness will increase as the real life tensions concerning failing health, mortality, and diminished life expectancies rise, unless these impulses to take satisfaction in things coming undone and falling apart are analyzed. This is not easy to do, and not only because raising the subject will arouse the resident's defenses, but also because, as part of these defenses, the resident will find it difficult to believe that they would be conflicted about their health and even about their mortality, but unless these impulses are given some way to enter consciousness they will only cause mischief and increase the human suffering of the resident, their loved ones, and the nursing home staff that work with them on a daily basis.

Before examining the unconscious and the preconscious urges to unite and to disunite, to come together and to come undone, however, and before examining the connection between these urges and certain representations of death in the unconscious of the elderly, I want to look at the nursing home as a social institution and as a social space where doctors, nurses, aids, and psychologists all perform certain roles and enact in the transference and the counter-transference certain unconscious urges toward integration and disintegration. For, although the people working in the nursing homes are for the most part caring, and indeed they perform work beyond the capacity of many, they often fail the residents on a deep emotional level because they react to their unconscious wishes, anxieties, hopes, compulsions about death and mortality, as well as their defenses and resistances without reflecting on them consciously. And, as a rule, nursing homes often are not equipped to address these sorts of problems because they see their primary purpose being the medical care of the residents and they rarely bother to inquire how their own unconscious feelings are affecting the level of care they provide to their wards. They, therefore, do not know what to do on an emotional level; and, therefore, they end up perpetuating institutionally sanctioned resistances to facing their fears and feelings as well as the feelings and fears of the residents concerning the place of death in their unconscious.

I base these observations on working with residents[1] in nursing homes for thousands of hours where I have seen first hand how the exposure to dying and mortality in the nursing homes reinforces a resistance to noticing the sudden and frequent rise in death drives among residents and staff. The danger that the death drive or one of its derivatives may become conscious sets off anxiety and defenses that take as their purpose to repress the signs of the death drive or to only allow it to enter consciousness if it appears disguised either as a symptom or by the defenses. This sort of resistance to acknowledging the place of death in the unconscious or this resistance to conceding its influence on the forms of care provided in the nursing home is an endemic problem in the care of the sick and the aging. And, one consequence of this resistance to addressing these unconscious anxieties is that modern medicine and the policy makers have not worked out how the elderly can live happy longer lives; and, in fact, many elderly people live poorer lives from a qualitative perspective.

In the coming chapters, therefore, I will explore these dynamics of resistance and defense in the nursing home settings from the vantage of seeing how it unnecessarily increases suffering of the residents, their families, and the staff. To properly set the stage, however, I want to make a few, brief comments on the new nursing home as a social institution and as a social space where men and women come into contact with one another; that is, I want to spend this chapter looking at the nursing home as a social space not only where the elderly go to live and be cared for at the end of their lives, but also as a place where their resistance to facing the place of the death drive in their unconscious is in full force This orientation will, I hope, provide a context for examining the relations between residents, staff, and family members as a psychological space where people relate, and do not relate, to the place of death in their unconscious and as a social space where people relate and do not relate to the ongoing clash between impulses to union and disunion.

Psychologically speaking, the nursing home has become one of the central places where residents, their families, doctors, staff, and so on confront their fears and fantasies about life, things falling apart, and mortality, even though this happens in most cases on an ad hoc basis or at least this happens in most cases at the level of people's unconscious and preconscious urges and defenses. One form that this resistance has taken is the near total dominance by medical discourses of the care of the elderly where emotional happiness and comfort are less valued than medical procedures. This has had both good and bad results, and, historically speaking, except for periods of epidemic, war, mass social dislocation or famine, the average length of life has increased markedly since the middle nineteenth century, but never so much as in the past thirty years.[2] Developments in modern medicine and in public health care largely explain this fact; which means that residents can live ten or twenty years in a nursing home. But, as we extend life are we also helping people face their death drives and the unconscious meanings they harbor concerning their death drive and their conflicted representations of satisfaction and guilt about it, or are we leaving them to face their unconscious and preconscious thoughts and anxieties about the fact that things seem to be falling apart alone? That the answers to these questions often are that we are simply not addressing these unconscious forces when we treat residents feelings is indicated by the fact that residents often produce a large quantity of death wishes that go largely unnoticed and uncommented upon; or that when a resident consciously expresses them they are treated as a suicidal patient and either over-medicated, sent to hospital, or placed under twenty-four-hour alert—that is to say, almost anything is attempted except exploring these thoughts and feelings, or, at least this has often been my experience while working in nursing homes.

The rise in death drives and the defenses against their entering consciousness are also due to the tension that is bound to arise when people's identity as nursing home residents clashes with their identity as members of a family. This tension occurs for the most part because the elderly have gotten themselves caught up in the expanding institutional power of medicine within the nursing home while the family has lost ground as the social space where the elderly end their lives. The day when sons, or most often daughters, cared for their ailing parents until they died is long gone. A staff of medical specialists and consultants do the health work now while most children visit mom or dad once a week, usually on weekends.

Nursing homes have become big business in the last thirty years, treating a wider population than just the unwell elderly. Today nursing homes also domicile people who need short-term physical rehabilitation and the chronically mentally and physically disabled who have nowhere else to go. But while these new populations are on the rise, the nursing home remains a social place where care and treatment of the elderly remains paramount and, as a result, even the care of the unwell but not elderly residents are impacted by the death drives that are stirred up in them by their own health problems and by their living in a social space dominated by the unwell elderly. Similar resistances, therefore, will appear in the unconscious representations and the symptoms of these other populations in the nursing home as well so that the entire institution becomes a social space where unconscious discourses surrounding death and dying affect all aspects of life and where the care of all the residents, whether they are older or younger individuals, will be affected.

While the nurses, doctors, and aides remain the backbone of the nursing home, today's nursing homes also employ large cooking and custodial staffs, social workers, recreational therapists, dietary specialists, and physical therapists. They also retain occupational therapists and consultants, including beauticians, ministers, priests, rabbis, and psychologists.

The psychologist occupies a strange, sometimes antagonistic and sometimes supportive, relation to other staff members in the nursing home. Due to the medical model employed in the nursing homes, the psychologist is usually a less important member of the staff than the doctor, and he cannot see a resident without the prior approval of a medical doctor. Also, in many nursing homes there is an understandable level of confusion, especially among aides but also often among the nurses, concerning the duties of the psychologist in relation to the psychiatrist.

As this suggests, the psychologist has to work around numerous difficulties that concern not only people's fear of psychology but which also concern the conflicting roles of various workers in the nursing home and their relative "professional" ranking in the nursing home's society. Therefore, if the psychologist wants to fit in enough to be able to do his job, he must remain flexible and inventive regarding the social rules and roles in the nursing home; and also he must stay flexible concerning treatment parameters, always bearing in mind he is not in his private office but is in a social setting with others who are not familiar with the index of psychology and its treatment parameters.

Sessions usually occur only once a week. The session time tends to be thirty minutes or fifty minutes but some residents need more or less contact. At other times, the main problem is finding a suitable space for therapy. Sessions often take place in the resident's room while another resident may be lying in their bed unable to move. At other times, the session may occur in a small examination room that is not an ideal space for therapy. Often there is a paucity of room so that staff resist having to give up a space once they occupy it. Sometimes a session gets interrupted because someone insists on occupying the room and a new space has to be hurriedly found. In one nursing home I had to fight with other staff for a month to get a room large enough for groups.

A second issue is the traffic on the floors. Noises coming from the hallway, other rooms, or over the intercom may interrupt the session. Unplanned hospital visits by residents may force the cancellation of a session at the last moment. Other events may conflict with the time of your session. The degree of coordination among staff varies widely between facilities. And unplanned family visits may force the therapist to change the time of the session at the last minute.

I treat more women (60 percent) than men at the time I am writing this chapter. While the average age of the residents ranges between 70 and 99 years old, around 25 percent are 40–70 years old. Ethnically, Jewish residents make up the majority (approximately 60 percent) with the remainder divided between Catholics (Italian-American, Irish-American), Baptists (African-American), Lutherans, or people who do not identify with any religious denomination. The residents come from all walks of life but the majority lived modest middle-class lives before coming to the home. Émigrés constitute a sizable minority.

Despite these differences, the residents have similar health problems. These include diabetes and the complications of diabetes such as amputated limbs. Some residents have become completely or partially blind from cataracts or glaucoma. Many cannot walk or walk with difficulty because of strokes, osteoporosis, broken bones, rheumatoid arthritis, or other chronic pain disorders. Respiratory disorders and chronic fatigue are common. Gastrointestinal problems, degenerative neuromuscular diseases, Alzheimer disease, vascular dementia, and other degenerative neural-vascular diseases affecting memory and thinking all appear frequently. Short-term memory deficits (especially new learning) are common, as are temporary states of confusion and impulsivity. The resident Axis I psychological diagnoses range from short-term delirium especially following hospital visits, schizophrenia and schizoaffective disorder to depression, paranoia, adjustment disorders or phobias. Many also suffer from underlying Axis II character disorders such as narcissistic personality with its characteristic grandiosity, lack of interest in others, and sensitivity to narcissistic wounding and borderline personality with its typical neediness, chaotic projections, unstable object relations, and relationships full of murderous *sturm und drang*.

The quality of care at the facilities varies. Two are very good facilities with broad bright clean halls and efficient staff. One looks out on a beach so residents can go outside on sunny days and see the ocean. The other overlooks beautiful rolling woodlands and includes a large indoor area where residents congregate and listen to music. A third facility offers equally good care as the first two nursing homes but does not look as nice since the building is older and less spacious. But it has its charms too. It faces a public park that residents can see from an outdoors area where many sit on warm days. The fourth nursing home has more problems. Each unit nurse runs her floor like a petty fiefdom and reacts suspiciously to outside interference. More importantly, the nurses do not always manage their units effectively. Orders do not always get written promptly. Residents sometimes miss appointments because the nurses forget to mark the time down on their schedules. And the nursing home often relies on temp nurses and aides who do not know the floors. These and similar problems have caused the Board of Health to inspect the home a number of times before my arrival. The administration let go a number of nurses and doctors in response to this investigation. But problems persist. It should be noted, however, that the state regulates nursing homes very closely and the home remains safe. Moreover, the shake-up has had some effect. The real problem in this and the other homes lies in the transference and countertransference dynamics on the floors, which is something we shall see again and again in the coming chapters.

To conclude, in the coming chapters I will explore how we treat the elderly in nursing homes and what role impulses toward union and to disunion play in shaping how these we relate, or do not relate, to each other when in these extreme situations. It, therefore, also brings the ways that the unconscious, and the place of death in the unconscious, shapes these good and bad interactions at the levels of emotional support that the elderly receive, or do not receive, in the nursing home.

NOTES

1. I generally saw residents once per week for thirty minutes or fifty minutes.
2. This is statistically speaking. There are, of course, groups whose birth and death rates have not followed the statistical trend for some or for all of the modern period.

7

Life for the Resident in the Nursing Home

The terrible foundations of Being are revealed.

—Nietzsche, *Thus Spoke Zarathustra*

In this chapter, I will explore the nursing home as a world of depression and envy. I also will show how these conflicts often occur unconsciously or preconsciously because of the defenses being deployed, precisely, to keep representations of death, dying, loss, and non-presence out of consciousness.

I became aware of these dynamics while working in a number of nursing homes in the city of X[1] where I noticed how frequently residents communicate unconscious and conscious death wishes, and behind these death wishes, if we take the time to tease them out, lay an entire, repudiated inner world of fantasies of dying or of other people dying, of things being broken or falling apart, of things being repaired and put back together, and of old remembrances of a destructive cast and of idyllic remembrances of things past.

Unfortunately, when residents arrive in the nursing home, they are already regressed and highly defended. They often come to the nursing home because they require round the clock nursing. In other cases, they arrive in the nursing home because they need short-term rehabilitation by medical specialists. Some come voluntarily. Often they arrive after consulting with children or because their spouse has stayed at the nursing home before them. Many, however, get there after a doctor orders short-term rehabilitation in the nursing home.

But whatever the circumstances that bring them there, residents soon find themselves forced to adapt to a society which creates a perfect storm for the arousal of old and new narcissistic fantasies of loss, of feelings the subject is on its own or has lost the object, and of feelings that the besieged subject finds itself in a threatening world where things constantly seem to be falling apart.

If we invent a "typical resident," we can imaginatively re-create what some of the external sources of conflict may be. Besides the obvious factors like health problems, recent losses, and so on, residents are forced to quickly adapt to a world where they give up much of their independence and many of the narcissistic gratifications they have fought to acquire over a lifetime. Our "typical resident" may arrive in the nursing home after having fallen at home or after a hospitalization. Initially, if he or she is elderly, they may experience a period of confusion. But even more alert residents may think that their stay in the nursing home will be a short one; and it may take them some time to realize that they are permanent residents if their rehabilitation does not begin soon enough or if the family does not, or cannot, take care of them. At other times, rehabilitation begins soon enough but then the resident falls or hurts herself in some other way that requires her to stay for a long time in the nursing home.

While our "typical resident" usually does not go to live in a nursing home until a health crisis forces her to have around-the-clock care, once she enters the nursing home, her daily life changes dramatically. While she may have lived in an apartment by herself, with a spouse, or in an assisted living facility before, she now gives up a good deal of her former independence and privacy. She eats when the aides serve food—usually in a common room located on each floor or alone in her room. She washes when the aides wash her. She goes to the bathroom when the aides take her, if she requires assistance. She usually lives in a double-occupancy room with another resident whom she frequently treats as an unwelcome intruder or stranger, although one resident I saw shared a room with a revolving door of short-term rehabilitation residents and another (many actually) demanded to be moved from room to room on a regular basis.

Thus, our "typical resident" must adjust not only to her own health problems but to living in a strange, and often inhospitable, environment. She often loses control of her finances. It goes to the nursing home or to a relative in most cases. More trouble usually follows. She frequently sells her apartment or home. This can create tensions and resentments with her children who usually are involved in the sale and it generally reinforces her melancholy over the loss of her independence. One resident I see lost her apartment when her family sold it after the death of her husband. Thus, while still in mourning, she had to adjust to the fact that she had nowhere to go and that she would spend her life in a nursing home. The anxiety and sense of her world coming undone that she experienced led her to symptomatic fears that the nursing home wanted to get rid of her too, and that she would have nowhere to go.

Thus, when they arrive in the nursing home, the everyday realities of life seem to conspire to raise the level of their discontentedness and resentment. The results are often what one might expect in this sort of environment: the resident rapidly succumbs to increasing levels of depression and this depression often centers on the loss of independence and pleasure-taking in life. The loss of self-sufficiency touches on other aspects of life, too. One resident who I saw for a number of years feels no pleasure in life because he has to eat specially liquefied food. Thus, our "typical resident" has to go through a grieving process where they mourn the loss of the independence that they struggled to acquire all their life and, at the same time, they also have to adjust to the reality of old age where they may no longer be able to do the everyday tasks they used to do.

Old age and life in the nursing home is likely to arouse old childhood resentments about having to do what the other desires, too. Many adults never develop very far beyond the comfort of desiring to satisfy the desire of the other anyway (initially, the desire of one's parents), but other adults spend a lifetime trying to create a psychological space where they can explore and, within the limits of their life, realize some of their own desires. When these sorts of people come to live in a nursing home, they may feel reinfantalized, and they may, consequently, resent the fact, for example, when they have to wear diapers again, lying in their own excrement because busy aides cannot change them, or when they have to lie in bed all morning waiting to be washed and dressed.

Very often, however, signs of a simple depression mask deeper unconscious representations of envy and the loss of the object. These representations of losing the object and feelings of envy stimulate inner representations of death and the struggle by Eros to hold things together. And this in turn helps sustain an unconscious culture at the nursing home dominated by the arousal and projection of representations of loss, of envy, and of the struggle to master the feeling of things coming undone. These largely unacknowledged conflicts, then, can spoil the inner happiness of and the communication between people visiting, living in, and working in, the nursing homes.

For example, the children of the residents struggle to master the anger and guilt that they can feel when they have to act as the parents of their parents because their parents cannot make decisions anymore. Such responsibilities arouse old tensions emanating from the child's own fantasy that its parent is immortal, but it also touches on their unconscious death wish for their parent, too. At other times it can arouse their unconscious representations of having been the object of their parent's death wishes.[2] These tensions arise because many children find that having to make life decisions for their parents that increase their parent's unhappiness feels highly guilt-inducing because seeing their parents reduced to a state of unhappiness arouses deeply ambivalent emotions of guilt and of feeling complicit in wishing their parents harm.

Usually, the children of the residents do not speak about their ambivalence voluntarily, but often it can be deduced by their erratic behavior, by their irregular visits, by the shortness of their stays, or by the angry, meddling way some of them relate to the staff. At other times, their ambivalence emerges in the way that they idealize the physician because they think the doctor will remove the burden of taking care of their sick parents from them. But when they do honestly talk about their feelings, the children of residents often express their profound guilt. Eventually, they will confess how disquieting the whole situation makes them feel. In some cases, fantasies and remembrances of being sent away to school and so on by their parents may emerge. They also may associate leaving their parents in the care of the nursing home staff with shadowy usually screen memories of their parents sending them away to some other "unspecified place," which we can associate to repressed representations of death, where death signifies "being abandoned and separated from the object" and of things falling to pieces.

Leaving a parent in a nursing home, therefore, will often elicit conflicting unconscious representations and emotions, including feelings of envy, guilt, and repair in the children of the residents; it also often stirs powerful, guilt-ridden feelings of relief at having gotten free of the burdens of caring for a sick parent day in and day out or of having to worry whether their parent may be hurt because of some oversight of their child or when they are absent and away. And, as I said, the act of sending a parent to a nursing home also often recalls repressed feelings of their parents having left them behind when they were children (just as Freud dreamt in the "Kitchen" dream that I reported on in chapter two).

On their side of the equation, the person left in the nursing home often expresses bitter feelings of having been left behind and abandoned; and, as a consequence, they often behave in an envious manner toward their children who they usually unconsciously, although not always, resent for leaving them when their visit ends. Their resentment often emerges after their children leave and it takes the form of anger or disappointment that their children do not visit them enough, a complaint that stirs repressed childhood remembrances in them of their own mother or some other adult not returning when they were needed; and it also stirs up their own guilt for having "not been there" for their children.

Sometimes, they also blame their children for taking their homes, their clothes, and their lives away from them, but for these complaints to rise to the level of a conscious complaint there usually has been a fairly severe regression on the resident's part or else there has to have been conscious conflicts and aggression between child and their parent for a long time; but, even in these situations, one is liable to find old repressed representations of being forgotten by the object, or of "dropping the baby," or some other guilt-ridden representation of things falling to pieces buried behind the signifiers of conscious anger and resentment.

Thus, very often, the smiles and happy faces that one sees when children come to visit their parent in the nursing home mask old and new unconscious representations of envy, of loss, and of guilt between the generations—and, the smiles may cover over ambivalent tension between destructive representations of things falling to pieces and other representations and defenses of things being put right and of loving remembrances; and, all things considered, the mutual envy and love binding the child to their parent is understandable. The envy that the elderly parent feels is especially understandable since it is partly stimulated by a real loss of independence and a real rise in unhappiness. For, when a resident comes to a nursing home she feels things have taken a bad turn, and this is bound to reinforce her representations of death and of her feelings of things going to pieces in her unconscious if these representations are not opposed by Eros.[3]

The most depressed residents wake up each day feeling more and more estranged and less able to perform the simplest tasks. She may feel physically sick and her libido may be drained by her loss of vigor; and, as her vigor dissipates further, she may spend most of her time in bed, or she may spend her time smoking outdoors or sitting in common rooms with other residents whom she studiously disregards. And, in general, although some residents adjust to their environment with little effort, and some even do emotionally bond with other residents, in many cases the residents who enter a nursing home discover that their desire for contact with others becomes shallower when it does not take a hostile form; and, as a result, many residents drift through the day, having lost sense and relevance, like K in Kafka's *The Metamorphosis.* As the depressed resident becomes more cut off from others, old repressed representations may emerge in her dreams and her discussion with the analyst that recall representations of having lost the object and of lack. Her life may be marked more and more by shallow erotic ties which cannot compete with the derivatives of the death drive in her unconscious. And, as a result, she may consciously feel empty and lifeless, or angry and defensive, her unconscious may be experiencing affective storms where she is exposed like the infant Oedipus to the elements to be eaten by wolves, or she may become like Jason who, in the end, came to see the fabric of his world unravel.

This is partly why the severely depressed nursing home resident so often feels useless; and it is also why she so often also begins to see herself as rubbish waiting to be tossed out rather than as a whole person. And, is it any wonder that she may envy her child for her freedom and youth, or that she may envy anyone else who has the gift of youth and the relative freedom and independence to get up and leave the nursing home? As one 94-year-old resident explained with great succinctness: "You're a young man. You work, have a family, and do what you like. For me [she makes a sweeping motion with her hand across her neck] the party's over." Then she repeats in Yiddish: "I'm just a big stupid nothing." An older Jewish man in his eighties who worked in a meat-packing factory most of his adult life simply tells me, "I ain't got any strength, no strength. I'm no good for nothing anymore," this coming from a man whose entire adult identity was defined by work and by putting food on the table of his family. Add to this the fact that work also satisfied old childhood desires to satisfy the desire of the Other, since in his mind so long as he worked he kept the love and satisfaction of the Other, and you can see that not being able to work carried with it an unconscious self-rebuke that he was no good to the Other anymore, too. Now that he could not work, the big Other would have nothing to do with him and he, like Samson, would lose his strength and wither away and, by consequence, was ready to be tossed aside, a feeling that he could not but associate to his declining health. His lamentations, therefore, reflected his unconscious shame that he was falling apart so rapidly that he no longer recognized himself, meaning that he no longer had a place in the scheme of things established by the big Other. I sometimes had the sense that he felt like those ancient heroes (Heracles comes to mind) who were cast out of the polis into exile, or perhaps a better description of his emotional reality would be to say that he is wandering the earth like old Oedipus bereft of the object longing for respect he no longer possessed, and waiting to die.

One hears Jeremiahs like this all the time in nursing homes. But it is a mistake to say that these complaints only reflect the depression of old age. To do so flattens out of a whole expanding space that signs of unraveling and the rising cathexis of objects by the death drive are taking up in the psyches of these residents.

Also, remember what I said in the first chapter about the formation of the subject. There, I wrote that the subject emerges at the behest of Eros to master the death drive and its representational forms. The simple diagnosis of depression, then, also disguises how much Eros has lost its ability to bind the death drive or to maintain the ban in the face of the growing disinhibitions of the death drive.

The nursing home is aware of these dynamics in its own way. What staff sees is that the resident appears depressed, anxious, disruptive, or noncompliant. And, they try to help the residents be more adjusted, happy, and compliant by providing them with entertainments and distractions. The home, then, does its best at trying to create a positive environment. For instance, they often have large recreation departments. They place prints on walls. They plan trips. They try to regulate the number of cigarettes residents smoke. In one nursing home I worked at, the residents play a game called Singo, a game in which residents guess a song after hearing a few notes. At other nursing homes people play bingo or they are entertained by often quite talented and hard working singers. And, for many patients, recreation proved to be a most helpful way of coping with their isolation and depression were it not for the fact that distracting people from their problems does not take the problem away for long.

Thus, the therapeutic benefits of distraction are often short-lived; and the resident is always faced with the fact that his problems return when the distraction has ended. In the long run, entertainment cannot remove the root causes of the resident's unhappiness, which include the fact that the resident does not want to be there in the first place and no Chagall prints or sea-view can make their health return or change the fact that they are living in a place where they fundamentally do not want to be living. Such a life is tailor-made to increase the quantity and the intensity of representations of death, loss, guilt, envy, and symptoms. Consequently, while they may adjust to the nursing home, they may not feel at home there; and, so long as this is the case, the chance of them feeling at home with themselves is unlikely, too. They begin to shut down and they cut themselves off from others who seem to arouse painful and overwhelmingly hostile emotions in them. These residents begin to avoid other residents and peer across at them with suspicion and derision in an effort to protect themselves from being too affected by others. A state of envy and guilt often overtakes them and spoils their relations to others in the nursing home, too. Of course, this is not the sort of situation that one only finds in nursing homes. All human relations involve frustrations that are liable to arouse unconscious fantasies of envy in people. But such encounters, which happen to everyone everyday, become exaggerated in the nursing home, which creates a perfect storm for the arousal of old death wishes and for the breeding of new death wishes, too. Also, envy, like the death drive itself, originates inside the resident's mind but easily comes under the influence of environmental frustration.

Thus, in one case, an anxious resident I saw shared a room with a woman who compulsively shouted "Can I get up now? Can I get up now?" and, "What time is it?" all day and night. For understandable reasons, the resident whom I cared for remained on pins and needles for the entire time they were roommates and she began to show signs in her conscious thoughts of rage and depression. She had a narcissistic personality to begin with, which only made living under these conditions even more intolerable for her. And, she began to show unconscious signs of envy that especially took the form of murderous thoughts and images in her dreams so that, ultimately, the best thing I could do for her was to strongly advocate that she be moved to a new room.

In another example, many residents sit in a common room with other residents where, inevitably, someone starts screaming in a way that many of the other residents find disturbing. This, then, can set off a shouting match between the screamer and other residents screaming back at her to "shut up." Apropos this sort of tit for tat shouting match, one psychotic resident in my care would regularly fantasize that aliens were tearing him apart when the shouting began. By representing his own rage and envy as "aliens who are assaulting him" this resident succeeded in transforming his inner psychotic feelings of being torn apart by his own death drive into a representation of an alien being who wanted to tear him into pieces.[4] In this manner, he succeeded in representing the profound disconnect he felt from the other, and which he only wanted to "obliterate" so it would stop persecuting him. Even non-psychotic residents, however, will project their fears that things are coming undone onto objects "outside of themselves" in order to turn hostile feelings inside them into an alien emotion originating in a "persecuting" other. And, in what at first must seem like a strange association, these feelings of unsafety often become linked to a feeling of boredom in the higher functioning residents who, in effect, manage their envy and fear of the other by masking it as boredom.

In carrying out this transformation of rage into boredom, the higher functioning resident is helped by the nursing home which can be an incredibly boring place to live. As I said before, many residents have nothing to do during the day but sit around. Lacking adequate stimulation, many residents drift in a sea of boredom. Boredom, however, has a secondary benefit for many residents who can be bored rather than become envious or anxious. Being bored, in other words, can serve internal processes, and play a role in the formation of a symptom just as well as it can reflect a deficit of external stimuli when the lack of external stimuli comes to signify a barrier against the drive to destroy the object.

Thus this deadening boredom, ironically, can become a last ditch defense against representations of death drives and anxieties entering consciousness or becoming too attached to the subject's conscious desires. For example, I treated a depressed eighty-eight-year-old man who smokes cigarettes when he can get them. While compulsively smoking, he obsessively complained to me about how bored he was in the nursing home. In one session after the next he complained that he could not wait until the nursing home organized a trip. This referred to the planned trips the nursing home organized outside the facility in the spring, summer, and fall months for the higher functioning residents. Residents who enjoyed these excursions gave glowing reports of having eaten dinner at this restaurant or seen that ball game. But while this resident dreamed endlessly of being somewhere else, he usually excused himself from going on these trips; and, although he would never admit it to anyone, least of all to himself, he really did not want to go on these trips at all; for, what he really wanted to do was to keep complaining and feeling bored because so long as he was preoccupied with being bored he kept his mind in a state of vacuous emptiness and like a postmodern Buddhist monk he did not allow his death wishes and anxieties the opportunity to enter into his consciousness.

He kept himself from being disturbed by his turbulent and unsettled inner emotions by emptying his mind of all stimuli; and, in an ironic twist, by obstinately not allowing stimuli to disturb his state of boredom, this resident succeeded in distracting himself from his own inner worries; and just like the idea of keeping the residents entertained, the path of remaining in a constant state of boredom followed by this resident ultimately ran into its own self-imposed limitation. For, behind his grumbling exterior this resident remained deeply, unconsciously disturbed and tormented by feelings that his life was coming undone and that he was being destroyed by his negative emotions.

In particular, his boredom masked disturbing unconscious remembrances and feelings of being "dropped" by his parents and then by life and in this sense, boredom saved him from consciously feeling he was being dropped again; but the price of barring these representations from consciousness may have been too high since it involved emptying himself of all comforting and comfortable objects, too. That is to say, being bored substituted one feeling of being dead (that is, he lives a deadening, boring life) for a worse one that his parents and the world had "dropped" him. Thus, by complaining that he has nothing to do, in essence, he succeeded in killing time rather than allowing the unconscious representations of his death drives to become conscious. But he had his limits. Winter is the cruelest season for him because the facility discontinues trips during the cold months of winter altogether, and, not surprisingly, his only outbursts, which included hitting residents, happen then.

Another elderly woman who lived in a nursing home, and whose unconscious was full of representations of wanting to die or to kill someone else, was only conscious of certain paranoid feelings that the staff wanted to get rid of her, although she could not say how and she concluded from her fear that her time in the nursing home was almost over, a feeling that had no basis in reality except as a projection of her death drive and as a distorted representation of her feeling that things were coming undone and would soon be over. She, therefore, ended each session with me by saying: "I will see you next week, if I am still here," which she meant for me to take quite literally.[5]

These symptoms had a specific motivation. They were designed to keep her from becoming conscious of her deep envy for her sons, and, although she could not, we can see her envy in a "happy dream" that she reported to me one day. In the dream, she had just bought a beautiful new apartment. When reporting the dream she emphasized everything was brand new and she also told me that she felt completely at home there. That was the dream she remembered in its entirety. I am taking the liberty of not relating all the associations to the dream that collectively pointed to a common idea that the "new apartment" expressed a wish both to get away from the nursing home where she definitely did not feel at home. But the dream also expressed an unconscious wish to be "young again" in the sense of everything being brand new!

A different resident, however, had a number of unconscious death wishes that were constantly threatening to break into consciousness. This is the resident who told me her life was over while making a slicing motion across her neck. And, these suicidal thoughts were quite serious. The defining event of her life occurred on her fourth birthday when her father departed for America and, ever since then she had unconsciously, and sometimes consciously, felt utterly and completely alone in the world. Being in the nursing home, therefore, merely reinforced a feeling of loneliness that had shaped her life ever since she was a child. In her sessions with me she sometimes discussed her wish to die, but this talk of dying was (in part) a ploy, for, she did not really want to die; or, at least, she did not consciously want to die, since all her real death wishes, of which there were plenty, were kept unconscious.

In her unconscious, loss meant "being reunited with her father" who, to her child's mind, she had driven away when she turned four. Thus, many of her suicidal ideas concerned her unconscious representations of having lost the object and already being dead, or else they concerned her defenses against these unconscious representations of absence and the loss of the object, but, not only that, many of her suicidal ideas concerned her unconscious envy that took the form of a repressed belief that she had driven her father away and, thus, that she had killed off the object herself. That is, her unconscious contained repressed fantasies of being dead in the existential sense of being completely alone after she had lost the object. Her grief then about being abandoned was worsened by her guilt for having "gotten rid of the Other." In this regard, her self-esteem was terribly injured and, finally, as a teenager, she had a miscarriage that she unconsciously experienced as a failed return of the object and the work of her envy; and, as a result, it quickly became another example of her murderousness.

Ultimately she could not escape her own persecutory impulses and fantasies. These and other frightening unconscious thoughts and feelings, however, rarely broke into consciousness as themselves. Rather, they appeared as a life-long depression that sapped the life force from her and symptomatically transformed her unconscious envy and signs of loss into guilty self-attacking thoughts like: "You wanted to get rid of me [the "father-Other"] so I left, but now you have to get rid of yourself!" This is one of the roots of her suicidal ideas.

The emotional effect this had on her was devastating, and this resident guarded her loneliness by repeating the act of emotionally killing off any representation of the Other that might wander too near to her. And people avoided her company to avoid her unconscious envy as a consequence. But, as I already showed, many other residents harbor envy for family and friends in their unconscious representations where envy is also bound up with signs of abandonment and loss of the Other, too, and with various other representations of the subject's falling apart and being destroyed. The woman who dreamt about moving into a new apartment can illustrate the association between envy and representations of the subject's experience of "coming undone" because her dream contained another wish that I did not mention before. Namely, the dream contained a fear that her sons wanted to get rid of her. At least at the preconscious level, they proved this to her by "dumping her in the home." The dream, therefore, presented her revenge against her unfaithful sons; for buying a new apartment and also meant having a new baby (as improbable a wish as that may seen for a woman in her eighties!), and by having a new baby, she also fantasized in her unconscious that she could get rid of those "good for nothing boys" by creating a new life. In this sense, the brand new apartment that would make her completely happy represented her having a new child. This dream also contained other envious wishes which in the best Machiavellian fashion implied that it was better to get rid of someone than to be gotten rid of by them; and, to refer back to the early discussion of her dream, it also alluded to the idea that you could always replace something old with something new and better. But, these feelings were present only in the unconscious because they would have horrified her if she ever became aware of them; and, therefore, instead of allowing them to enter consciousness, she felt disquieted and guilty.[6]

All these examples point to the same direction: they point to the conclusion that residents struggle to repress their unacceptable feelings of lack, envy, guilt, and revenge. To refer to just one more example, a resident that I saw on Saturday sat anxiously in the waiting room for me. When I approached her, she nervously said that she was waiting for her daughter who she expected at any minute. Since it was already 4.00 p.m., this was highly unlikely. When we explored what had happened in a later session, she said that she became overwhelmed by fear that her daughter was never coming to see her again, something that objectively was not true, but was a true expression of her unconscious envy.

As the frontline of the nursing home, it was often the staff that got the brunt of the resident's envy and resentment for having to do what they were told to do. Hence, for instance, residents complain that the staff harbors them ill will. And, these feeling are only partly projections; for the staff, by necessity, bring their own unconscious envy and guilt to their job. And we would expect nothing less, given that working in the nursing home stirs their mixed emotions about aging, mortality, and death, too.

The staff's job, including appearing caring when they feel mad or resentful, creates a large amount of latent aggression in them that tends to come out in their relationships with each other and the residents,[7] and, as a result, the interpersonal relations in the nursing home are often dominated by resentment and envy even when everyone is trying to do their best to get along. The situation is worsened by the fact that the staff is not emotionally trained or prepared to deal with all the thoughts and feelings that come up in their jobs. Some aides and nurses, for example, yell at the residents and other staff on days when they feel overwhelmed by the demands of their job. But passive aggressive behavior is a far more common reaction to the build up of aggression among the staff. Many aides, for example, only change the resident's diapers at predetermined times like a mother who only feeds her baby on a fixed schedule instead of when their baby feels hungry. Other aides and nurses do not acknowledge residents calls to change their wet beds because they feel the resident is too demanding or because they feel the resident asks to be changed too frequently.

One distraught resident complained to me that her vagina had discharge and that she needed to see the GYN but that the nurse ignored her requests. When I asked the nurse, because the resident's complaints are often distorted and exaggerated, she said that the resident just saw the GYN three weeks ago, so, if she had an infection it must be because the resident had "dirty hands." Obviously, such egregious behavior is not the rule and is not acceptable but even where the behavior of the staff is far more humanely professional one still finds outbursts of rage, envy, and guilt that muddy the relationships and may lead to the crossing of emotional boundaries that cause things to go all wrong and end up badly; that is, one finds boundary violations that cause the dynamic in the nursing home between staff and resident to slide into a state dominated by investments in their death drives followed by equally self-destructive narcissistic defenses, as occurred, for example, when one aide told another aide—without a bit of irony—how she never let the aides in the nursing home where her own mother lived wash or dress her: "I do everything. I wash the cloth, make the bed, and I feed her," she added, because she did not "trust those aides one bit."

Thus, as this aide knew all too well, kindness in the nursing home can screen more hostile intentions. Residents can be fully aware of this, too, as occurred, for example, when a resident with brain damage causing him to substitute sounds like "boom, boom, boom!" for emotionally charged words spent a whole session complaining about a disingenuous nurse who, he kept repeating, said to him: "My, don't you look nice today!" but who really meant, he said: "I do not mean it; I'm just pretending!"

There are numerous cases like this when the staff turns their hostility against the residents without realizing what they are doing. For example, doctors and administrators who ration medicine to save money may also be rationalizing cruelty without being aware that they are being anything but responsible, good members of the "health care team." Likewise, doctors who spend most of their time reviewing charts and writing orders rather than making rounds sometimes also illustrate how institutionalized care often run at the behest of the insurance companies can be too dehumanizing, especially when doctors know a lot about the resident's medical conditions but very little about the residents as people.

As this line of thinking suggests, regulations and a standard of professionalism will only go so far in helping the staff respond to their unconscious guilt and envy. This means that a professional attitude may help stabilize group identity and provide the staff with the means to measure their productivity. But when following professional rules and guidelines serves as an end in itself, it tends to increase the staff's latent hostility. Thus, following professional routines assures that pills get dispensed in a timely fashion, showers happen on schedule, and that meals get served on time, but it does not prepare the staff to deal with the complex emotions that their work arouses in them. Of course, this is not always the case. I have worked with very caring staff who take time to know the residents they treat. But, at the same time, one cannot deny the fact that some professionals wish that residents would psychologically "go away" so that they could get on with the business of treating the disorders in the chart or staying on schedule. And, it is for this reason that everyone would benefit if staff were taught to explore their fears and fantasies about death and if they received training in how to recognize transference and counter-transference feelings. And, beyond simple training in how to recognize projections, transference, and resistance, the staff should be encouraged to see that residents are suffering from the ebbing of their Eros and the rising tide of their death drives.[8] And, apropos this, the therapist remains charged with the task of helping residents and the staff establish new libidinal attachments to the therapist and to each other and face their conflicts regarding mortality.

All this is necessary because the nursing homes can create a perfect storm for the arousal and defense of unconscious envy, guilt, and anxiety; and, as a consequence, the staff and the family who visit their parents in the nursing home will be invested by their own unconscious and conscious envy and depression, too. Many people feel deeply narcissistically that all their efforts to achieve some autonomy and to realize some of their own subject's desires are falling to pieces; and they begin to feel anxious, angry, sad, and envious as a result—something that will further arouse old resentments and representations of having lost, or being about to lose, the subject's symbiotic or special Imaginary connection to the Other. As a result, many of the people I have discussed here have severe narcissistic disorders that have either been caused by or have been worsened by the decline of their health, the loss of loved objects, and the threat to their mortality. Conflicts around death wishes—things like representations of unconscious envy, representations of unconscious guilt, unconscious representations of death, anxieties that the subject is coming apart, and opposing representations that things are being repaired and that the subject is being put back together or that the subject is magically resurrected, that is, that the subject is magically immortal—can be seen in the tensions that arise in resident's children, too.

In the next chapter, I will explore how some of the staff and some of the residents in a nursing home defend themselves against their death drives differently. In particular, I will show how some of the staff may try to disavow the need to mourn, or to accept their fear of dying, while some residents may try to negate their envy of the dead.

NOTES

1. I am basing these observations on thousands of hours working with approximately 65 residents a week in four nursing homes where I treated more women (60 percent) than men at the time I wrote this chapter. While the average age of the residents ranged between 70 and 99 years old, around 25 percent are 40–70 years old. Ethnically, Jewish residents made up the majority (approximately 60 percent) with the

remainder divided between Catholics (Italian-American, Irish-American), Baptists (African-American), Lutherans, or people who did not identify with any religious denomination. The residents came from all walks of life but the majority lived modest middle-class lives before coming to the home. Émigrés constituted a sizable minority. The quality of care at the facilities varied. Despite the differences, the residents have similar health problems.

2. The impulse to deny their emotional conflicts attempts to keep them from facing painful affects. Very often these primitive mechanisms, whereby the resident tries to free himself from his negative affects, are sustained by powerfully active unconscious fantasies of being immortal, sometimes replete with childhood fantasies that they had magical powers to conquer death. Immortality fantasies like these often are located at the base of the resident's defenses, so that it becomes difficult to determine in some cases which came first: that is, it becomes difficult to decide whether in the defensive system the resistance emerged from a childhood fantasy of invincibility or, on the other hand, whether the fantasy of being able to survive death (to stop things coming undone) was a byproduct of the resistance—a fantasy that the subject needs to create to help it believe it is not in danger when it is in fact surrounded by dangers. One sees, I suspect, that the Achilles heel of this piece of magical thinking lies in the inescapable fact that denial, and not noticing what is happening, only goes so far before reality returns and upturns the whole idyllic lie.

The problem, then, is to figure out what to do with the death drive and the pain associated with it. Should we continue to try to repress them and then deal, in a rather blind and ad hoc manner, with the consequences—high anxiety, regression, defenses, and the formation of symptoms that mirror the unconscious conflict without acknowledging it? Or, do we try to make the residents loosen their resistance a little and modify their defenses so that they are not instinctively repressing the death drives so much and so that they can make the unconscious source of their symptoms more conscious?

3. Very often the resident's reality testing at first works against their ability to master the derivatives of their death drive. For, if she cannot accept her new life graciously, then, it often is because she knows that (for the time being and maybe for the remainder of her life) she will lose a great deal of independence.

4. His belief that he can defeat the aliens (in an intergalactic battle after the world ends) reflects the continuing influence of his weakened-but-not-all-gone Eros which still opposes his death drive and forces it to veer from its ultimate aims.

5. Another depressed person with dementia who has lost both his legs due to diabetes tells me that the aides in the common room are discussing who they will kill. When an aide opens the door for a second to the room in which we were talking, he adds that she has just come back from a funeral and then, after asking me not to be frightened, tells me that she came in to see if we were dead. When I asked him why she would do that, he replied that whenever aides open closed doors and peer in they are checking to see that no one is dead. When I ask him what they would do if they found us in the room dead he says that they would cry and then bury us: "There nothing to be done about it," he concluded.

6. Her dream was, therefore, partly an erotic dream of seduction that did not get discussed as part of the transference analysis.

7. When working in such an environment, it is only human that the staff would at least, in part, respond to their own death drives (where they encounter so much falling apart and coming undone) and that they would also respond to the death drives of the other staff and residents in ways that are full of magical thinking and defenses.

8. Only a love not dominated by destructive impulses can help the resident to resist falling into depression, extreme anxiety, or despair. Therefore, the first job of the psychologist is to listen to the typical ways the resident represents, in his own life-history, the urges to disavow the death within and to transform it into something external and threatening.

8

Residents' Narcissistic Frames of Mind

> A strong egoism is a protection against disease, but in the last resort we must begin to love in order that we may not fall ill, and must fall ill if, in consequence of frustration, we cannot love.
>
> —Freud, "On Narcissism"

In this chapter I want to suggest that we think of the depressed mood that is so prevalent in the nursing home in a different light than we normally do. Instead of treating the depression of the residents as a chemical imbalance of the brain or as diagnostically self-explanatory in the first instance, I want to focus on what is happening to the resident's sense of themselves as a subject in relation to the Other while they live in the nursing home. And, in particular, I want to argue that what we describe as a depression can also be described as the gradual withering away or collapse of the subject's attachments to the Symbolic order as their old ties to the Symbolic world are, one by one, broken; and as a result of the loss they are experiencing "the shadow of the object falls across the ego." I will, at least for the most part, hold off on analyzing the simultaneous collapse of the subject's relation to the Imaginary other until the next chapter. But I will, at least, want to set this collapse on the subject's Symbolic ties to the Other in some sort of context with the simultaneous collapse of the subject's Imaginary ties to the Other as well. For both separately and in combination partake in a more general psychological catastrophe in the lives of many of the residents.

To begin with, the sometimes gradual, and sometimes rapid, unraveling of the subject's Symbolic ties to the Other is only the first act of what can be seen to be a three act tragedy. In the second act, as the ties binding the resident to the Symbolic world wither away, their subject falls into stages of Imaginary loss and merger with the repressed maternal Other. In this second act, which corresponds with the growing isolation and separation of the subject, we find a number of merger fantasies, a growing number of anxieties, as well as envious fantasies. And, then, finally in the last act, as the break with the Symbolic order has advanced quite far, and as the grandiose and narcissistic conflicts surrounding the Imaginary have become more pronounced, we find a growing preponderance of fantasies and anxieties concerning the possibility of the subject simply collapsing into "nothingness."

This then is the general itinerary that the resident follows: it is an itinerary that is also a retreat back into an identification with "nothingness" by the subject and I mean to equate this fantasy of the subject's collapsing into "nothingness" with the fantasy of the nonbeing of the subject, of its death as a subject or as a subject who is coming to identify with imaginatively rushing toward its own nonbeing rather than being a subject who creates structures of desire to hold this experience of "nothing" at bay. But to begin with, I need to make a few preliminary comments on what I mean by a person's "narcissistic-frame of mind" in relation to the subject's Symbolic, Imaginary, and Real ties to the other. In the first instance, we need to distinguish the narcissism of the ego from the subject's narcissistic ties to the other. Afterward, we also will consider the narcissistic disorders of the self. This is a difference few took notice of before Lacan, and, for most of the history of psychoanalysis, when the analyst spoke of narcissism, he or she meant to refer to the ego's narcissism, or the libido's investment in the ego. But, additionally, by narcissism analysts often mean a developmental stage associated with pre-oedipal life. In this sense, a baby, even if they are born object-relating, is also born narcissistic, and that baby remains overwhelmingly narcissistic in its object choices for many years before it is able to relate to other Symbolic allies as separate from itself. Winnicott's concept of the transitional space is surely central to this process of separating out, and then coming to relate to, the other as a part of a "not me" world. So, too, is Peter Fonagy's, Mary Target's, et alia descriptions of mentalization and how children build up an inner world. And so is the build up of inner models of attachment and separation in the development of the mother-child dyad developed by John Bowlby, Margaret Mahler, Fred Pine, and many others. But so too, finally, is the subject's coming to relate to the other through the medium of castration anxiety in the oedipal conflict and beyond.

But to stress the developmental component of narcissism and the gradual build up and solidification of a subject's relation to an object world does not mean that an adult who has already built up a rich inner world with secure attachments and self-object representations cannot still be dominated by primitive narcissistic fantasies and defenses, especially in their ego's unconscious representations. Either as a result of fixations or regression, one can speak of a narcissistic relation to the object, as Freud does in "Mourning and Melancholia," where he describes libido reinvesting the ego with the longings and hate it felt for a lost object. In this definition, narcissism is a defense against the loss of the object and the rise of aggression that gets turned against the ego in melancholia and in the mourning process.

Also, a primitive narcissistic frame of mind is not the only kind of narcissistic frame of mind one is likely to encounter in people. Narcissism is not only a primitive state that is eventually given up for an other-oriented one. Instead, narcissism develops and there are states of more mature narcissism. The development schema of narcissism cannot be reduced to a choice between love of self (narcissism) and love of others (object oriented libido). The fact that the ego is itself built up from "lost objects" and introjected Others belies this. Also, the ego develops from more primal into more mature forms; this was something that Lou Andreas-Salome stressed in her work in the 1910s (to Freud's approval) and which underlies the whole self and object-relations universes, so that the individual is able to relate to itself and to others in more or less secure ways. Thus we can speak about egos which are secure not only in their attachments to others but also about subjects and egos that are more secure in themselves.[1] We also have to bear in mind that there is a descriptive definition of narcissism too, which can be summed up by the phrase that a person is "self-centered." This is what people usually mean when they say that "X is narcissistic," and it is in this form that narcissism has come to be related to other negative signifiers like being "conceited," "self-absorbed," and "full of oneself." But, people also speak of narcissism in a similarly descriptive but positive ways, too. Thus, narcissism, in the sense of self-love, can become "a protection against disease." Freud often spoke of the prophylactic function of positive self-regard. And others have concurred that positive self-esteem helps a person face life's ups and downs without collapsing into sickness. And, we know, for instance, that positive self-regard can strengthen the auto-immune system. Hyman Spotnitz et alia have argued, for example, that the person who does not hold onto his anger is less likely to contract cancer, and other specialists have studied the health effects of positive self-regard for the management of pain.

Thus, it is a mistake to limit a discussion of narcissism to a "disorder of the self," as some psychologists do; but it is as grave a mistake to speak of narcissism only in regards to the primitive ego.[2] For, as I have said, and as is already widely acknowledged, the persistence over time of primitive, narcissistic defenses is also associated with powerful, poorly controlled representations of the death drive in the unconscious and it also is associated with the formation of powerful, poorly controlled symptoms of death and dying or of things being destroyed and falling apart; while, at the same time, developing mature defenses and forms of narcissism helps the mind to control these death drive representations and these symptom formations of the death drive; and it also allies narcissism to the aims of Eros more successfully.

We have become so acclimated to hearing phrases like "falling to pieces" as being the same as phrases like "schizoid anxiety" that we often forget that it is also a definition of the urge of the death drive, too. Or, we can speak of the self, the subject, or the ego's feeling itself united with a greater power which is capable of swallowing it whole, like the white whale swallowed Ahab in *Moby Dick*. Similarly, Lacanians can speak of the Real, Imaginary, and Symbolic registers of narcississm, and can equally refer to the ways that the three registers get "knotted together" and come apart.[3]

To keep these definitions separate, but also to see how they may be related to each other, think of the first definition of narcissism (I mean the developmental one) as a higher order definition that expresses the changing ways in which the life and death drives are being represented narcissistically across the life span of the individual. Alternatively, we can think of the Real, Imaginary, and the Symbolic registers as expressing the three dimensions of narcissism at the level of representation of these underlying drive conflicts (of repetition compulsions, traumas).

I think that, bearing the distinction in mind that the ways of relating to the drives narcissistically can be placed on a structural and a developmental scale clarifies the narcissistic condition in some way.[4] We also should bear in mind that, for Freud and Lacan at least, there is an important distinction between primary narcissism and secondary narcissism that bears on many of the complications I have been alluding to in this chapter, and which Elisabeth Roudinesco explains in her essay "The Mirror Stage: An Obliterated Archive" when she writes that: "Primary narcissism is a first state, prior to the constitution of the ego and therefore autoerotic, through which the infant sees his own person as the object of exclusive love—a state that precedes his ability to turn toward external objects. From this ensues the constitution of the ideal ego. Secondary narcissism results from the transfer to the ego of investments in objects in the external world. Both primary and secondary narcissism seem to be a defense against aggressive drives."[5] What Roudineco suggests is that primary narcissism is somehow equivalent to the Mirror Stage when the ego and the subject both come into psychological existence through the child's identification with the spectral image of its "fully coordinated" and perfect body. Thus, on the one hand, the sort of narcissistic disorder that Freud describes in "Mourning and Melancholia" would in this schema refer to the secondary form of narcissism when the "shadow of the object falls across the ego." And, as the quote at the head of this chapter implies, Freud always felt positive self-regard to be barrier to illness. But at the same time, he believed that narcissism is not enough since the ego needs an object to keep from falling ill. For the subject needs the other. And, the latent link between Eros and health can be seen in the way that too much narcissism is a sign of illness and will eventually lead the individual either to unhappiness or ruin. In the domain of sexuality, this is, I believe, one of the lessons Freud wished to be drawn from the primal murder myth and, ultimately, from the dual drive theory itself, where anything that weakens or limits Eros will eventually accrue to the advantage of the death drive. Similarly, Lacan drew our attention to a similar fact by different means. For, if Roudinesco is right about the Mirror Stage, then one can conceive of the Imaginary as an effort to avoid taking the step toward object relations by, in essence, leaping over the object and by only having one special other, finding in oneself a universe that needs no other. In short, the child finds itself in an "exclusive relationship" captured by the maternal gaze and made manically "whole" by the mirror.[6]

Initially then being captured by the gaze of the Other constitutes the subject's narcissism on wholly libidinal and erroneous grounds. The child constructs the image not only of the maternal gaze, but a maternal gaze in which it sees itself reflected not as it is, all uncoordinated and needy, but as it would appear in its ideal. Thus like the Freudian baby who fantasies the absent breast to calm itself, the Lacanian baby enters a world of fantasy satisfaction when it enters into the Imaginary. And, just as the Freudian baby who hallucinates the breast is bound for disappointment that will drive him forward toward a new confrontation with the Real, so too the Lacanian baby's ideal image of itself is bound to crash against the limitations of fantasy. One final thing I hope to show is that a good deal of the narcissism of residents originates in primary narcissism; that is, it originates in the experience of losing the primal object of desire: something that already is illusionary image that is designed to plug up the hole of a more primal "nothingness."[7]

In stressing the importance of distinguishing the narcissism of the ego, the self, and the subject, I do not think I have said anything more than what people already know. Also, I think it is fairly common knowledge that narcissism can be spoken of in senses other than the ones we have spoken of so far, including ways that bring the association between narcissism and the life and death drives to the foreground; that is, narcissism can also be spoken about in a sense where narcissism, in both its primitive and developed forms, can represent a manifestation of Eros and the death drive can take in the mind. In this regard, one can speak for instance of narcissistic injuries in which the mind feels it is about to fall to pieces.

Having provided this short, and barely sufficient, introduction to the rather complicated subject of narcissism, I am now prepared to launch into a discussion of the pathologies of self-love of a number of nursing home residents in the following pages of this chapter. To begin with, the reader must remember that residents' self-esteem is often deeply bruised by the time that they reach the nursing home. Many have lost spouses, are sick with severe heath problems, and feel pushed aside by younger family members or by the other symbols of the big Other in their life. But I have discussed all of this before so I will limit my comments to saying that these and other factors cause many residents to be emotionally battered when they enter the nursing home world and already well-versed in the loss of objects that define the narcissistic disorders of the self and secondary narcissism.

One resident, for instance, describes her fellow residents and the staff as completely undependable characters who want to persecute her. The other residents and staff are, in her view, contemptible, and she avoids them as much as possible so as not to throw pearls before swine. She separates herself from them whenever she can and adopts a queenly insouciance toward them most of the time. However, her narcissistic grandiosity masks a real narcissistic battering caused by the loss of the objects in her life.

Her narcissism, which can be described as a defense against the loss of the object needs to be distinguished from this form of narcissism. Narcissism rooted in envy often plays an increasing role in the mental life of many residents, too, and it often may structure their conscious and preconscious attitudes toward life and death. Thus, when a resident's sense of envy is already well-established in their psyche, the wish to get rid of it uses their preexisting pathways. The following set of associations made by another resident illustrates this point. After a violent hitting incident against another resident, she told me that she tried to not think about dying, "but it comes to my mind anyway." Her associations then turned to a further thought which summed up her belief that: "Everyone dies, even the Rockefellers and J. P. Morgan." And, when she said: "Even the Rockefellers," she meant to say even *the rich and powerful* (which is one class she envies) die. In other words, this resident managed the anxiety aroused by the representation of her own death wish by turning it into a statement of envy turned against the rich and powerful because she finds this form of aggression more acceptable to her superego. Her superego even allows her to feel some pleasure in the bargain. She grinned briefly as she did away with the Rockefellers in her imagination. And this had the added bonus of converting her initial anxiety into a pleasurable death wish acceptable to her superego, while, at the same time, inhibiting her impulse to go into action by hitting someone. The displacement of her death wish onto a suitably contemptible object, finally, kept her own death wishes from ever reaching consciousness.

The logic of the displacement was from a death wish directed against herself to a death wish in the disguised form of envy for some loathsome other. A dangerous impulse to die was substituted by another one that has the following structure: "I should not die, but those rich and powerful people who are really no better than me should die," where those rich people are to be understood to include the class of all people she envies, including the other residents. And, not only does she displace her anxiety into envy, she then adds a consoling moral platitude to please her superego as an afterthought: "You see," she adds, "God is fair to everyone. Everybody dies," meaning, everyone deserves her envy. "Sometimes," she concludes, "the rich die sooner than others."[8]

A useful way of conceiving this is to see that this resident's ties to the Symbolic world are collapsing while her archaic ties to the most primitive imagoes of the mother are reemerging to disturb her consciousness. Thus, her depressive withdrawal from others is being driven by the break of the social ties that normally protect the subject from its own archaic ties to a primitive envy where the role of the other recedes further and further into the background. If we explain her regression in this way then we can begin to see that she is doing more than falling into a depression that causes her to withdraw from others, because her withdrawal is accompanied by unconscious paranoid fantasies of destroying the other qua object and of being destroyed by the Other, that in some way, given the paranoid structure to her desires, rises to the level of consciousness.

There is a link, then, between the depressive withdrawals we encountered in some residents and the rise in paranoid regressive states that occur as the resident ties to the Symbolic, and the whole Symbolic world appears to be failing the resident. For as the Symbolic ties to others begin to break down, the collapsing world of the Symbolic can no longer adequately shield the subject from knowing the extent to which the whole chain of signifiers is sustained by a repressed castration anxiety. A marked increase in castration anxiety and conflicts around the defense of the subject from knowing that it is ground in lack appear. So too does the anxiety surrounding the Imaginary merging with the "phallic" maternal imago, and this increases the conflicts relating to the falling to pieces of the ideal, the "problem of object loss" and "schizoid anxiety" which are so well worked out by the object relations school.

This collapse of the Symbolic is precisely what has happened to the resident I discussed earlier, whose father went away on her fourth birthday, except that in her case there appears to have been a general failure of the

Symbolic order from the start of her life that severely disturbed not only her Imaginary ties to the Other, especially the Other represented by her absent father, but also severely undermined her subject's capacity to find adequate Symbolic substitutes or even to develop ways to signify stable attachments to objects. The subsequent losses that trigger a failure of the Symbolic order for other residents merely reinforced her already preexisting sense of the failure of the Symbolic order to help her escape from her Imaginary entanglements. Having never entered the Symbolic order in a secure way, this resident's desire only developed as a paranoid structure where the price of encountering the Other (her father) would be catastrophic for her.

Apropos this, Freud, who lacked the language of structural theories of desire developed in the fifties, sixties, and so on, wrote in *Beyond the Pleasure Principle* (1920) that the deepest source of resistances lies in a compulsion to repeat painful traumatic scenes in which no pleasure seems to be derived from the act of repetition, but only a mechanical compulsion to repeat can prepare the ego for the return of the trauma—and, this is what we see occurring in the mind of this resident whose whole mental structure is based on the subject remaining tied to the Other in some fashion.

This uncanny and unsettling relation to life is central to the world view of Kafka's characters, too; and, as such, it is obviously not restricted to the elderly, but forms a part of the general trauma, the truth of desire that simply occurs with greater frequency in the nursing home, and which, Freud told us nearly three-quarters of a century ago, is defined by a compulsion to repeat which remains "beyond the pleasure principle." That is, it remains on the other side of the pleasure principle and is, like some "barbarian Germanic tribes" of ancient Rome, from the perspective of the Romans, somewhere "beyond the pale." Thinking of residents as being in the midst of a traumatic relationship to life and to the traumatizing collapse of the Symbolic ties to the Other often extends to the residents' fantasies of their bodies which seem to have been handed to some sadist. Thus, many residents at one time or another refer to their own bodies as if they were not a part of themselves. Hence, they talk of how "it" shits and pisses; "it" assaults or betrays them with "its" pain and diseases. This relationship to a persecutory body-self resembles the schizophrenic fantasies that Victor Tausk analyzed in the patient he encountered in a sanitarium who thought her body was a "desiring machine."[9] And, in fact, I treat schizophrenics who imagine their bodies are machines of torture or machines of war. In some cases, the boundary between word-representations and body image has almost completely broken down so that they experience fantasies as if they are sharp or shooting body pains. We are encountering minds for which the Symbolic shield against Imaginary persecutory fantasies has almost completely collapsed, and, similarly, we are encountering minds in which the boundary between drive and representation itself has become nearly obliterated; and, increasingly, this body-speech marks the spot of a mechanical return to a trauma in which the resident's body seems to them to be going through a process of disintegration or coming undone. One resident who suffers from painful arthritic knees cannot think of anything but her pain for days at a time. Her pain signifies her mind's assault on her body. And, these preverbal pains bring to mind past anxieties of her stomach cancer and the loss of her parents when she was four years old.

As in the case described above, many residents feel pain at a preverbal narcissistic level at which point any emotional contact may become too much for their thin stimulus barriers; such residents experience even the slightest disturbances as a gross over-stimulation that threatens them with rising death drive derivative. In such cases, the balance between the life and death drive is tilting drastically toward death, and the supply of Eros is dwindling dangerously low. In these cases, regression threatens to invest word- and body-images with primary narcissistic terrors which usually emerge at a preverbal level of body pains and which also emerge in the presentation of images and thoughts of the subject's coming undone. Often this force is so powerful or persistent that it simply overwhelms the ego, leading in some extreme situations to death or to the eruption of death images into consciousness. This happened with one resident who returned from the hospital having lost the will to live so completely that even staff, which was oblivious to such things most of the time, saw it was just a matter of time before she would lose all hope and simply perish. Her condition did decline rapidly, for no apparent medical reason, and she died three months later.

In these extreme cases, narcissism becomes less a defense and more an agent of the death drive. And, this is a very different reaction than we find in residents whose withdrawal from the external world succeeds in strengthening their stimulus barrier. In other cases, a good prognosis can be made even with severely withdrawn residents if they are capable of holding onto transitional objects, be they pictures, a wedding ring, or even stuffed animals, because this ability to remain attached indicates an ongoing connection to something besides themselves (so, too, does a relationship to family, staff, or other residents). In one case, I worked well with a resident whom the staff found "impossible" because I knew she could still form attachments when I saw the dolls that her husband had given her during their years of marriage neatly arranged on her window sill.

Behind the emotional struggle of some residents in the nursing home lies the clash of the drives and, because of this, even severely regressed residents can strive to hold the death drive at bay a little while longer by narcissistically investing libido in things. It is into this struggle that the analyst makes his or her presence felt by "containing" the resident's feelings of falling to pieces, and by providing safe enough conditions for the resident to begin to relax some of her resistances and to replace some body symptoms and representations of chaos with words, and, finally, by allowing new structures of desire binding subject to the Other to emerge out of the catastrophic collapse of the old Symbolic and Imaginary forms of desiring. By using the degree to which a resident regresses to, or fixates at, a narcissistic frame of mind as one measure of the resident's mental strength or deterioration,[10] the most dangerous situations can be confronted together.

According to Angel Garma, "traumatic neurosis" defines what occurs when a large quantity of stimuli floods the mind and overwhelms it. And, we can already guess what this means in the case of many residents as they slide to a condition where over-stimulation comes from the clash of the dual drives. At this level, it is sometimes vital to reinforce the resident's secondary narcissism, even its illusory qualities, if the only other alternative is a decline into the conflicts of primary narcissism. At least secondary narcissism protects the residents from deeper trauma. One sees this shift from a relatively stronger secondary narcissism capable of holding the death drive in check, toward a still ambivalent longing to merge with the big Other and so to die, to rest as Shakespeare wrote, in cases like the Czech resident who while waiting for her father's return turns what seems like a case of secondary narcissism with the shadow of the object having fallen across the ego into a defense against the total collapse of the Symbolic order itself that, in her case, turns waiting into a masochistic longing to die. But all is not lost either, for, by fantasizing that God does not love her enough to let her die, this poor resident manages to raise her terror of "nothingness" to a representational level and so maintains some Symbolic distance from her inner trauma. Thus, what started as a defensive "I want to die" masking a hidden desire to be with her father again slowly became a struggle to maintain some distance from her wish to "nothingness," which is for her impossible, by making death the final victory of her fantasy that she will be reunited with him only in death.[11] The end result is a sharp rise in the representations of self-destructive impulses (in the guise of unrequited love) but no real suicide attempts.

In sum, I have argued that there is a connection between developmentally primitive states of narcissism and increases in death drive activity, especially in forms like a rise in representations of envy. This rise in envy often is accompanied by a slide from a state of secondary to a state teetering on the conflicts of primary narcissism where the Symbolic order seems to collapse into a terror of "nothingness." What is breaking down, then, is not only the ties forged by Eros and the Symbolic order but the resident's ability to form non-Imaginary identifications. Besides the real loss of external supports and the death of loved ones, therefore, residents are often thrown into a terrifying regression. Severely disturbed residents are plagued by the general collapse of the Symbolic order, and this makes many of them fall into a paranoid, archaic relation to the maternal imago where the subject has no ballast against her deadly *jouissance*.

In other words, the resident slips back to the Imaginary anxiety of not existing, that is of not being a subject or an "I" at all. To not function as an "I," or rather to have to function in this "I-less" way, means that the individual has lost all relation to the world and has collapsed into primary narcissism and is at risk of being totally swallowed up by the Other-death. When the resident loses this sense of "I" then she finds herself well along in a process that ends in death. That is why the loss of the sense of identity of residents, like the older man who worked in the meat packing factory all his life, is so much more serious than it may seem at first. And that also is why to diagnose such a person as only suffering from a depression that can be treated psycho-tropically is to grossly misread the traumatic event that may be occurring in that man's psyche. For, the mind's collapse toward primary narcissism not only will arouse terror by itself, but it also will stir up ancient, primitive anxiety states that date back to the oedipal complex and to the child's painful separation from the time when the structure of desire was exclusively Imaginary and Real but had not yet become Symbolic—this is, to the time when the subject and its desire had not yet been made an object of exchange and Symbolic substitution, before it had become linked to the world of object relations.

As the structures of desire collapse there is, first, a rise in "castration anxiety" and the various other forms of anxiety that Freud told us are unified into the single sign "castration" in *Inhibition, Symptom, and Anxiety*. These include birth anxiety, separation anxiety, and death anxiety. But as the Symbolic collapses further the subject becomes more exposed to the "impossible" terrors of the Imaginary surrounding merger, the collapse of the ego ideal, being swallowed by the Other, and ultimately falling into "nothingness" which the Symbolic fear of "castration" had replaced.

The Symbolic order, at least, with all its limitations, provides the residents an unconscious set of relations to make sense of the impossible contradictions of their lives and gave the child a way beyond the "impossible" desire for the mother and the "impossible" demands that the mother's *jouissance* placed on the child's structure of desire. In essence, language saves the child from this "impossible" situation. It establishes a Symbolic universe in which desire can circulate beside lack, where one signifier can act as the subject for another signifier, and ultimately where every signifier can stand in for the signification of the subject of castration and nothingness. All signification fills in this gap, this nothingness. The price the subject pays is high—castration anxiety. No matter what, it can never replace or refind the primal fantasy object but only finds counterfeit satisfactions that can only reinforce the ultimate despair of finding the lost Thing. All that remains is to either remain stuck in this impossible quest for something that is not even real or to embrace life on its own impossible and incomplete terms (these are the terms that language has imposed on us).

Neither desire nor the desiring subject is ever stabilized so long as it remains trapped in the fear of "nothingness." This can be seen very clearly by spending any amount of time with residents in a nursing home. For, having lost their jobs, their connections to loved ones, and to a shared life, these residents find their sense of identity so severely threatened that life and the demands of, and desire for, the Other appear more and more meaningless. A vicious decline begins, a slide into the conflicts of secondary narcissism followed by a fear of collapsing into the conflicts of primary narcissism, so that the further the resident regresses, the stronger their death drive will be.

As the subject slides back toward primary narcissism, on the drive level, the resident's Eros begins to weaken. The great fear is of "nothingness." A situation that recalls Lacan's famous image of the Imaginary register in *The Four Fundamental Concepts of Psychoanalysis* (1964); that is it calls to mind Lacan's image of a vase, where the vase itself is the Imaginary image which captures and encloses an interior space that is only "empty space." Being has no form in the way empty space has none, until it is enclosed by the image. Later, while revising Freud's oedipal complex (which he called "Freud's myth"), Lacan will explain how the Imaginary form of desire is slowly abandoned by the child who, following the hints of the mother's desire, turns to the father and the Symbolic order for a new structure, one in which an "impossible" desire can be endlessly replaced by objects that never quite succeed in capturing or enclosing the whole of the lost, original, "impossible," desire. No secondary form will succeed in capturing what could not be contained even in the original image. In essence, the vase is supplemented by the Law of castration whose purpose is to allow the child to separate from its exclusively Imaginary ties to the maternal world.

It is the reversal of this telos (or perhaps a better way to say this is that it is the completion of this telos since all arrows shot into the air rise and then fall down to the ground again) that plagues the inner lives of many residents; a reversal by which the subject's way of relating to the Other becomes dominated more and more by eroticized death drives, and where it is the loss of the Symbolic world that will precipitate the crisis and the fall down to the conflicted world of exclusive maternal imago and "nothingness."

In this state of affairs, narcissism becomes the last refuge of Eros for those who are on the slippery slope between life and death. In this sense, narcissism becomes a final defense that fails since, by withdrawing their last attachments from the world and giving them narcissistic investitures, residents succeed only in cutting themselves further and further off from supplies of Eros and love that, as Freud writes, are the only things that can in the long run keep them from falling ill. And, as their withdrawal from objects proceeds, they increasingly adopt more primitive and extreme pre-oedipal defenses like projective identification and splitting to manage their aggression and feelings of loss.

It has been my experience that when patients are in a severely regressed state, their minds are more likely to become more narcissistically self-destructive and to generate destructive representations of dying and death, or of things falling apart, a fact that the Kleinians and the British Middle Group understood in their discussion of patients' primitive "schizoid" and "psychotic" rages and in their talk of the mind's terror that it was "falling into bits." From our perspective we can say that minds experiencing the sorts of "psychotic fears" that their mind or body would fall into bits are representing the conflicts of primary narcissism. But these conflicts are not being expressed in a direct manner but are instead translated to the level of representations and drive compulsions to repeat the slow decay of Eros and the victory of the death drive over time.

What the analyst needs to do in these situations is not only provide the resident a container to "dump" the *jouissance* of the Other and the *jouissance* localizable in their own body. Rather than simply being a container, the analyst also needs to provide secure and dependable boundaries for the resident who is being threatened by the collapse of the old Law.[12] Like Oedipus, residents are likely to already have had the veil lifted from their eyes in a way that has traumatized them.[13] All that is possible, then, is to help them retain whatever hold they have on their own desire and to help them to finally guide the ship of their life to its final destination peacefully, to help the residents finally disentangle themselves from their desire for the desire of the Other and to acknowledge that all their debts to the Other have been more or less paid. I plan to explore one or two more cases of death fantasies and the other fantasies of escape and repair in more detail in the following chapter.

NOTES

1. These later ideas have been taken up by different schools including the attachment theory school (Mary Main et al.) where the focus remains on the development of secure attachments to the other and Heinz Kohut's self psychology school which

emphasizes the development of a secure inner representation of the self-object (but, again, through internalizing a secure self). Heinz Kohut, *The Restoration of the Self* (Chicago: The University of Chicago Press, 2009); John Bowlby, *Loss: Sadness and Depression (Attachment and Loss)* (New York: Basic Books, 1982); Peter Fonagy, Gyorgy Gergeley, Elliot Jurist, Mary Target, *Affect Regulation, Mentalization, and Development of the Self* (London: The Other Press, 2005).

2. Then, of course, there is the Lacanian perspective to consider. For Lacan, the "self" is not the equivalent of the "ego," that is, the ego is as an illusion and resistance; or the Lacanians speak of the ego as being a construct of the Imaginary register, which, for Lacan, comes down to the same thing since the Imaginary is a kind of illusionary register where the ego forms out of a fantasy of the self as whole and coordinated as the "man in the mirror."

3. Thus, psychoanalysis, in particular, has stressed the connection between early childhood trauma, fixation on early narcissistic failures, and the prevalence of powerful, destructive representations and urges. Kleinian and British object relations theorists, for example, have focused on early "schizoid" states where the mind feels all split up and "falling to bits"; and, from a drive theory perspective, these representations can be seen as the representations of the clash between Eros and the death drive, in which the ego is being overwhelmed by fear of dying and of things falling apart.

4. This is similar, in some senses, to the difference between (multiple) synchronic and diachronic (or even between structural and new historical).

5. Elisabeth Roudinesco, "The Mirror Stage: An Obliterated Archive," in *The Cambridge Companion to Lacan* (Cambridge, UK: The Cambridge University Press, 2006), 96.

6. We see here the difference between the object and the Other. The object is the substitute (to use a Marxist term) fetish of the Other that contained the child's original "impossible" desire.

7. In her essay on the mirror stage, Roudinesco uses this felicitous way of putting this: "In abandoning himself to death, he seeks to rediscover the maternal object and clings to a mode of destroying the other that tends toward paranoia." Roudinseco, "The Mirror Stage," 114.

8. This resident is typical in that she suffers from a rise in death drive activity and a decline of the quantity of Eros capable of opposing it. For her striking out is an expression of her thought that "everything is falling to pieces" and that the social bonds are frayed and coming undone. The resulting rise in tension in her causes her to regress to even more primitive, narcissistic projections. She hits, in other words, partly because of the rise in death drive investments of her narcissism and in part to put a stop to them by projecting them outside of herself.

9. See Roazen, *Brother, Animal: The Story of Freud and Tausk* (New York: Transactions, 1990) where the Tausk-Lou Salome-Freud triangle is discussed and the article is cited.

10. And, as a general rule, the more nearer to primary narcissism, the more the resident struggles with her fears of dying; and the greater the quantity of representations of death will appear in consciousness or in the preconscious as the subject teeters toward death.

11. Illness influences the ebb and flow of Eros and destructive impulses in the mind in ways we are just now beginning to understand (at least on a neurochemical level), but are far from understanding adequately. The brain connects to every part of the body, including the immune system, the parasympathetic and sympathetic nervous system, and the endocrine glands. The whole body is, therefore, connected together and the neurochemical balance in the brain affects how we feel, think, get sick, and heal, and vice versa. But the mind is not simply a passive observer of things happening to the body.

12. If time permitted, the analysis should help the resident see that the Law and the subject's relation to the Symbolic order is itself ground in illusions (or constructs of language). But under these extreme conditions, the analyst is best advised to help the residents hold onto the Eros that they have.

13. I am of course referring to the Oedipus at the end of "Oedipus Rex" not the wayfarer Oedipus found in "Oedipus at Colonna."

9

The Negation of Death in the Nursing Home

In this chapter I want to examine a number of defenses against making the death drive accessible to consciousness. I actually plan to look at two defenses, one commonly exhibited by the residents and the other commonly exhibited by the staff in the nursing home. In both cases, I want to argue that the defenses allow the staff and the residents to deny or disavow their powerful, negative emotional investments following the death of a fellow resident in the nursing home. Then, I want to follow this up by exploring a poem by Allen Ginsberg precisely because the poem is about how we mourn or do not mourn in ways that do not hide the terrible reality of the loss of a father but that also do not exploit it for melodramatic purposes or use it to bring life to a halt. That is, Ginsberg's poem tries to put death in its "right" context, which is "nothingness," and so helps his readers see how to manage their similar grief at the loss of a loved one. Finally, I want to refer to some ideas found in the writings of Freud and Lacan on the status of nothingness and the death of the subject that also allude to a number of their comments concerning how to face death and "nothingness."[1]

I think the easiest way to understand these defenses is to start with a "typical" occurrence in a nursing home: the unexpected death of one of the residents. When residents and staff learn of the recent loss of fellow resident X, they react like a person in shock. They pretend nothing has happened, or they acknowledge the death only in whispers and then try to put it out of their minds as quickly as possible.

Thus, when X dies, a wall of silence descends on everyone. The removal of X's chart may be the only concrete indication that he has passed away since this means that 1) a doctor, administrator, or nurse is reviewing it, 2) X has gone home or to some other facility, or 3) X has died. If I ask someone what happened to X they may tersely tell me that he died. Or they may disregard my question altogether. But their demeanor will betray their anger that I have mentioned the thing no one is mentioning. At this point, I know that the conversation has ended. If I push on, however, and ask how X passed away, I usually receive a curt reply like age, complications, or something equally unenlightening, and this really ends the conversation for good and all with everyone going on about their business very much as they had before.

What does this wall of silence signify? Perhaps it illustrates people's sense of delicacy. There really are, after all, social rules guiding how we should react after a recent death. There are thing we do not say to this person or to that person. And, there are things we simply do not do. But, in this case the delicacy of the staff is not socially sanctioned, although it does bespeak a certain preconscious group-think about how to manage the delicate period immediately after someone dies in the nursing home. Silence generally reigns on all the floors without any intended "consensus." The best explanation for this silence is a psychological one: according to this explanation, no one wants to dwell on something so disturbing to the general functioning of the nursing home.[2]

But, the important thing to bear in mind is that this defense arises from a visceral need for the subject to deny its emotional investment in nothingness and an equally visceral need for the subject to deny its emotional investment in its own "nonbeing" (Freud's aims of the death drive). The defense, in other words, allows the staff and residents to know but simultaneously refuse to take notice of the fact that a death has occurred, or that this death is stirring unpleasant, and sometimes aggressive, associations in their preconscious and unconscious thoughts and feelings.

The need to negate the death of X, then, includes a need to not stimulate nearby aggressive associations which can instead find expression in a variety of projective mechanisms and in a higher than normal level of depression.[3] The staff must negate not only their feelings about X, but also, they must negate any idea of their own mortality or the mortality of those they love stirred up by X's death. For, if it is not closely guarded, X's death may become a stimulus for a cascade of other associations to past and present object loss; whereas, by negating the idea of death, the staff hopes to simultaneously negate and "cut off" any association to its own experience of object loss, too. What most concerns the staff, then, is 1) to not arouse their superego by allowing anxiety to enter into their conscious minds (in this sense, they are resisting feeling guilt) and 2) to not arouse their own destructive id impulses, or the representations of these id impulses (thoughts and feelings about their own death and the death of those whom they love) by thinking about X's death. Thus, by disavowing their feelings about X's death, they shut down their guilty and anxious pathways; but they do so at the cost of producing a minor distortion to reality.[4]

This sort of distortion of reality can best be described in the following way: Even though everyone knows X is dead, and that everyone will eventually die, the staff proceeds as if nothing occurred which might disturb the ongoing life of the nursing home. In this sense, the individual is symbolically "sacrificed" for the peace of the whole.[5] Thus, the staff collectively and individually knows but does not know. This is the classic definition of negation given by Freud in his famous 1925 essay "On Negation," and, in particular, the defensive version of negation where reality is being avoided and disavowed.[6]

Thus, the staff simply withdraws a certain amount of its collective libido from the thought of a resident's dying in their midst and uses it to reinforce their ego which has experienced a potential loss; and, in so doing, the staff compensates itself, and protects itself from any supplemental anxiety that has not been completely negated by the experience. And, in line with this defensive function, the staff proceeds as if it does not know, and in this way removes "something unpleasant" from its experience of reality, and spares itself the pain of an object loss.

Thus, when faced with death, the staff experiences a collective form of magical thinking; and, while in that state it behaves as if the death of X simultaneously can be acknowledged and negated. And this is a little bit like a child pretending that bad things do not or did not occur or a child pretending that they did not wish X to "go away" in the past. The other side of this magical thinking is the equally fantastic belief that only those whom you dislike and so turn into strangers actually die; and this belief certainly offers a powerful explanation for the hostility the staff sometimes shows to residents, for it is only a small step between wishing to negate X's death and wishing X dead.

These various self- and other-directed destructive impulses, however, also come out in the cruel behavior I described earlier. Let me offer just one more example as a reminder. Once, when I went to see a resident who has a diagnosis of bipolar I disorder, I found her sitting on the floor in the dining room. At least four or five aides are there. So too are about twenty other residents. When I ask why the resident is lying on the floor crying for someone to help her up, an angry aide barks at me that she is a "manipulative one." When I say that howsoever that is you cannot leave a resident in tears on the ground, I am told that they have gotten her off the floor twice and each time the resident fell back down. "She can just lie there for a while" another aide says. Such inexcusable behavior stems from a sadistic wish which remains split-off and negated to punish the resident for stirring up unsettling anxieties about dependency and death in the staff.[7] But this and similar forms of acting out by the staff of its collective aggression is the other side of an impulse to negate the death of X.

But the residents show no more desire to explore their feelings about the death of a fellow resident. I only recall one resident inquiring about a dead resident: "You see," this resident confided to me, "we were friends and no one will give me an answer." On one other occasion, a resident expressed grief for a recently deceased fellow resident. "We sat at the same table together," she said, and "he folded napkins for me. Who will look after me now?" These confessions of loss, however, were exceptions that proved the rule. In general, residents exist in states of desperate isolation and they are too obsessed by their own problems to acknowledge the passing of another resident. This means that their grief is normally directed toward themselves more than toward any recently deceased resident.

Thus, although they too studiously disregard the loss of others, the resident's reaction to X's death reflects a different relationship to life and death than the staff. For, while the staff enacts a fear of death and a refusal to mourn, and therefore to acknowledge, their own mortality and the mortality of those they love, many residents show a growing hatred of life which is simply the consequence of living with so much pain and sadness for so long for which they take larger and larger quantities of drugs, and for which their lives seem devoid of happiness. They feel as if they no longer control their existence. Many know that they only have lived as long as they have due to the interventions of modern medicine. And this explains a great deal of their hostility toward doctors and staff. In this state, many wish for nothing more than to die, and they look on any steps necessary to keep them alive by staff as sadistic. Indeed, one reason they avoid thinking about X's death is that they do not want to acknowledge their envy of the dead.

Up to this point, we have examined two responses to X's death. The staff's reaction demonstrates the strategy of refusing to mourn. This failure to mourn, however, leaves them cut off from their feelings and vulnerable to split-off anxiety and violent affects that they project onto the residents and other staff. Residents do not have the luxury of refusing to mourn in the way the staff does. Instead, they try to not think about X because they do not want to become too aware of their envy of the dead. But this leaves them vulnerable to further regression and to the return of the violent death drives they wish to keep out of consciousness. Both staff and residents, in other words, respond symptomatically to any sudden rise in death drive activity or any sharp increase in tension states due to the clash of this drive and the countervailing urge to deny death.

We know, of course, that the thing that cannot be completely said is the extent that the ego is identified with death and the "necessity" of living in a reality distorted by castration anxieties. This repetition of a trauma, including castration anxiety, to keep a wish to die from becoming conscious suggests that without the trauma in the mediated form of the repetition compulsion coming between us and death, we would be likely to simply disappear in into Heidegger's "river of becoming." And, in fact, some people do succumb quite easily to the failure of Eros to hold death at bay and deteriorate into inorganic components of life.

Another, more structural way to imagine this is to say that the ties binding the subject to the other are cut and the subject itself is "no more." Ferenczi makes a similar point while writing about his treatment of RN, an intelligent woman who had been sexually molested as a child. Ferenczi writes: "I know . . . that there can be frighteningly painful moments, in which one feels one's life so appallingly threatened, and yet oneself so weak or so exhausted by the struggle, that one gives up. In fact, one gives oneself up."[8] Ferenczi goes on to add as an allegory the following account:

> As an analogy I refer to a reliable account of an Indian friend, a hunter. He saw how a falcon attacked a little bird; as it approached, the little bird started to tremble and, after a few seconds of trembling, flew straight into the falcon's open beak and was swallowed up. The anticipation of certain death appears to be such a torment that by comparison actual death is a relief.

Thus, it is the envy of the dead who feel no more tension about staying alive, and the anxiety aroused by this envy, that the residents want to disavow when they split their perceptions of the death of X. And, like the staff, they avert their eyes while the procession of the dead pass them by, since what is at issue is not acknowledging the extent to which they envy the dead having escaped the struggle of life for good having entered a final state of rest, an end to suffering, and a return to Heraclitus' river after such a long time.[9]

In short, what is given up in this situation is the desire to live, and, for this to happen, the ties binding the subject and the other have to be broken. This ambivalence between dying and denying we are going to die lies behind one resident's fascination with birds. An east European Jew, he spent the war years fighting against the Nazis with the partisans; for most of his adult life since the war he has mastered survivors' guilt by opposing it to his pride in fighting in the resistance. His ability to willfully push depressive thoughts out of his mind is the most striking aspect of his personality, and like the music of one of his heroes, Beethoven, he forces himself not to sink into depression, and instead to remain alive and creative. Apropos this, he once told me that he spoke with his sister on the phone. "She sounds not so good," he reflected. "I prescribed that she spend more time with young people. But she does not agree. What, she told me, would young people have to say to an old person like me? I disagreed, of course. You must struggle against such feelings."

In our first session, he showed me photos of himself after the battle of Berlin, which he participated in with a group of partisans and soldiers attached to the Polish army. "I am a soldier," he quietly said in that first meeting. Among his activities in the nursing home, this soldier-survivor feeds the birds with which he has established a very fond relationship. Not all the birds, however, have won his affection. He prefers the small sparrows that swoop around him while he throws them bread crumbs. But when a bigger bird approaches, one of the many seagulls for example, he stomps his feet and growls until they fly off because he defends the little guy. His relationship with the sparrows also reflects his ambivalent attitude toward life and death as well to the extent that, like Beethoven's ninth symphony, the sparrow will rise higher and higher in flight, expressing a mounting tension between two competing urges and images. One is of vitality conveyed by the image of the "soaring sparrows," but the other is a preconscious image of the dead souls of the crematoria and battlefields flying away to heaven, as well as a desire to reunite with them which he resists.

We are clearly beyond the pleasure principle and into the experience of a repetition of a trauma, but a trauma in which one side is committed to disavowing death and the other is drawn to it. Such sudden rises in tension and death drive activity, of course, are unavoidable in nursing homes. Aging and the approach of his own death only intensify these tensions.

As a being in which being becomes partially conscious, humans are existentially and psychologically torn between the urge to return to the death drive and to treat it as a foreign and dangerous seduction. But for the most part, this war within remains unconscious, and it creates a second front where the defenses try to keep the state of tension caused by this inner-war out of consciousness as much as possible. In these encounters the defenses are trying to restrict its entry into consciousness and only allow it to pass in the guise of a symptom.

In sum, under most conditions, the last thing residents want to do is think about X's death because 1) his death threatens to reveal the extent to which they all have sunk to states where the tension caused by the need to struggle with the death drive breaks into consciousness and 2) because, precisely for this reason, the residents secretly envy X for having escaped the trauma of being. That is, he has escaped from the need to exist within a Symbolic world in which relations are based on castration anxiety and the demand to disguise the fact that so many relations contain a fear of castration. And, of course, one finds the struggle to carry on and resist the drive to return to nothingness occurring behind these castrating structures of desire. Similarly, a good deal of the staff's hostility toward residents can be lain at the feet of their inability to mourn and the staff's magical wish to 1) relieve themselves of undesirable guilt and anxiety and 2) to reaffirm the Symbolic order that they, as medical workers, ambivalently still represent.

In both cases, a defense will be used to negate or deny the effects of that inner struggle to postpone the terrifying encounter with "nothingness," or, if you prefer, the terrifying encounter with "absence." Each type of negation illustrates the mind struggling to keep something unsaid or unfelt; it also reflects the mind's increasing inability to carry out this wish in the face of failing health, old age, and death. Thus, in the final section of this chapter I want to turn to the topic of religion, poetry and "nothingness." For, not long after the death of his father, the poet Allan Ginsberg wrote about what we do following the death of a loved one in which we have a different response to grieving "nothingness."

Indeed, since we are speaking now of the loss of a father by a mourning son, we have reason to believe that Ginsberg had good reasons for wanting to defend himself against the pain and scarring of death on the human soul. And, yet, Ginsberg wonders if we can find a space for nothingness in our daily living. Or, does death—or any severe trauma—simply overwhelm and shatter our normal existence?[10] There are various ways to read this poem. In one, Ginsberg wants to change our normal associations to death. Death will only signify "nothing." This is the Buddhist form of nothingness which sees all representations of suffering and desire, including our fear of loss and nonbeing, as illusions and as aspects of the world of Maya, and, therefore, of no more consequence than a fly buzzing around our nose as we meditate on the illusion of false attachments (that nevertheless cause us so much pain). Yet, Ginsberg's poem can be read in other ways too, even though they may go against the intent of the poet. A different reading maintains the tension between our ironic and paradoxical longing for a state of nothingness and the real pathos of personal loss by trying to understand how suffering has made us the people we are and how it continues to define who we are today. The result of this approach to nothingness may, ultimately, come to "nothing," since focusing on the structure of our desire may make us less attached to things—especially less attached to the desire of the big Other—but we shall see.

In general, life contains many forms of suffering, and the subject can find itself in many different structures of desires; thus, it does not help bring us nearer to the Real if we define suffering simply as an illusion. I am not saying this is what Buddhism is advising us to do; for one thing I am not an expert on Buddhism which, in any case, has many contradictory schools, like all religions do. Rather, I am speaking of an illusion that can infect Buddhist teaching, just as it can infect any form of desire, which states that if we could only just not suffer then we could see life unclouded by our subjective obsessions. One epistemological version of this position is the idea that if we just put our subjective feelings to one side we can somehow see the problems of life objectively—that is, not as it seems to us to be but as it really is beyond our subjectivity.

This position, of course, involves magical thinking originating in the operation of the pleasure principle, which, in fact, is not the agent of the Real so much as it is an agent of the imagination and pleasure-seeking. To approach the Real,[11] the mind has to, first of all, enter as deeply as possible into its own subjective experience of suffering and of pleasure in order to discover how the world symptomatically appears to it[12] as knotting (tying) the mind together into forms that replace the repressed *jouissance* of the body and the struggles between Eros and the death drive to destroy and to unite.

For example, we see a general withdrawal from the world in depressed residents that the DSM-IV R manual associates with things like anhedonia, apathy, isolating behavior, rises in anger, and so on, but which also describes the state of desire that the subject finds itself in as its identifications to the Symbolic order are falling to pieces. One expects this to be a highly painful and disturbing process as the resident experiences one loss after another and one Symbolic cord after another is snapped. And, after this process has progressed quite far, we do see a general collapse in the subject's relation to the Other and to images and illusory forms of wholeness and completeness which are the other side of the body's loss of coordination as the residents go through amputations and diseases that all contradict the subject's "special" Imaginary relation to the Other.

Thus the collapse of the Symbolic order is followed, and accompanied, by a collapse of the Imaginary world as well that belies the real uncoordination and ravaging of the resident's body and his emotional life. The rise in Symbolic castration anxiety, which is the other side of the subject's defensive effort to hold onto his Symbolic ties, is therefore accompanied by a rise in defensively produced imagery of the wholeness and completeness of the subject, too. But, the fall into a world of Imaginary fantasy and defenses ultimately cannot defend the subject from the subject's real fear—a feared collapse into, and fantasy of, merging with "nothingness."

Remember, Lacan represents the way the Imaginary and, later, the Symbolic, order functions as a defense against the subject's fear of collapsing into "nothingness," when he spoke in 1964 of the Imaginary as being like a flower vase which surrounds nothing and replaces this nothingness with "something," namely the vase itself.

In the first instance, this image of the vase surrounding nothingness is an image of the maternal (Other) surrounding nothingness, of being, but it equally is an image of the subject who is joined to the Other, and merged with it, against the terror of non-being. And, the terror of non-being is the ultimate fear of the residents in their regressed states: they fear collapsing into "nothingness," into the same nothingness that Lacan reminded us, in the same 1964 seminar as the flower vase image, that the Imaginary baby fears when it fears the non-presence of the Other. For, ultimately, it is the Other (the maternal imago in the first instance) who guarantees life and stops the subject's fall into nothingness and non-being. And thus, it is the fear of the Other's non-presence that arouses the fear of falling to pieces and of coming undone that Freud taught us is the aim of the death drive in *Beyond the Pleasure Principle* (1920).

This fear of death, and the premonition that all humans have of their own mortality, leads them to fantasize a world beyond death. But these illusions, like the subject itself, are developed to create a barrier against the wish to die. And, to the degree they are agents of Eros, it is the wish to die and later to murder that the entire mental world (the structures of the Real, the Imaginary, and the Symbolic) are set against. Ultimately it is this double fear—the fear that the subject will collapse into nothingness and the fear of the subject's own desire for death—that preoccupies the residents in the nursing home, as their Symbolic and Imaginary ties to Other give way to a growing desire to merge with "nothingness."

Thus, the Imaginary defense against merging with nothingness finds itself full of "holes" and gaps that let the desire for nothingness come through. In such extreme situations, even the repetition of a trauma may defend the ego against nothingness and, in essence, hold back the rising tide of the death drives; for, even a trauma in the mediated form of the repetition compulsion can come between the subject and death, and the subject's submersion in the flow of becoming. In essence, the elderly are losing the form of a living subject and deteriorating into the inorganic again.

Another way to express this is to say that the process of developing the structures of desire in order to repress the desire to return to nothing begins to reverse itself. Thus, even though the child's world is saturated by Symbolic meanings and structures that he cannot comprehend from birth, from a genetic perspective, a child passes through a Mirror stage first before identifying the structure of its desire and the formation of itself as a subject in relation to the Symbolic order. In essence, what occurs at the diachronic level of maturation of the individual is this: at first the child's subjectivity and desire are constituted around an Imaginary axis until eventually the "impossibility" of the child's capturing all the mother's desire leads it to follow her lead and start to desire the Other of the Mother. That is, the very nature of desire, that it cannot be satisfied completely and to the exclusion of the desires of all others, leads the child to seek to "find itself" and to locate the satisfaction of its desire in the Symbolic order. This, of course, casts the subject (Heideggerians may prefer to say "throws the subject") in an "impossible" quest to satisfy its own desire in a linguistic universe where all the signifiers are ironically, tragically signifiers precisely because they refer to the one signifier that is both excluded from the chain of signification, and makes it possible by being its negation, namely the Name of the Father, which is the signifier signifying castration.

The price the child pays for identifying with the Symbolic order is the foreclosure of its original desire (for the mother's exclusive desire) under the threat of castration. But at the same time, the subject finds itself upon a path where, whether it remains in the Imaginary or Symbolic level, all signifiers ultimately signify and cover over the subject of "nothingness." The price one pays for not falling into nothingness is to remain in a world of desire in which no desire is completely satisfying or hits the mark. This is partly because the mark is itself an illusion of the desiring subject to cover over the knowledge that no object can replace its primal desire. In this sense, one can say that behind the Imaginary and the mother lies "nothing."

One consequence of this, according to Lacan, is the notion that "castration means that *jouissance* must be refused, so that it can be reached on the inverted ladder (or inverse scale) of the Law of desire."[13] One way to read this, and it is one I suggest we take seriously, is that Lacan is saying exactly in relation to *jouissance* and desire what Freud is saying about the relation between the life and death drives in *Beyond the Pleasure Principle* (1920). Namely, he is saying that the direct route of the death drive must also be refused, so that it can be reached on the inverted ladder of Eros and the law of castration. Or to say this more simply, the aim of Eros is to reach the state of inorganic rest, but only after the possibilities of Eros have all been exhausted.

But to return to the previous example I had been developing, it is by separating from its original desire that the child-adult sets out on the lifelong journey to rediscover the lost object of desire in a substitutive form. It is therefore one of the ironies of Freudian drive theory and Lacanian theory of the formation of the subject of desire that in both cases, life in the case of Freud and desire in the case of Lacan is a long detour from one state of nothingness to another. Moreover, for both Lacan and Freud, it is a question of Eros and desire reigning itself in, failing outright to realize their primal goals, and limiting itself to forms that escape death by excepting the possibility of castration that makes life and desire possible.

Apropos this, the Lacanian analyst Alenka Zupančič argues that for Lacan castration is a different notion than it is in the work of Freud being that when Lacan speaks of castration he lays the stress on the structural role that castration anxiety performs in keeping the *jouissance* of the mother from overwhelming the subject. Castration, then, writes Zupančič, protects the child from the terror of being swallowed by *jouissance* of the Other, of literally becoming nothing. Hereafter, to the extent that the subject's desire for the Other is regulated by Symbolic exchanges, it will live within the tyranny of the Law that is also a defense against the collapse of the Symbolic back into the terror of being swallowed whole by the maternal imago. However, as the Symbolic and the Imaginary orders fail, the superego becomes more paranoid as the Lacanian subject and the Freudian ego simultaneously align themselves more with the aims of the death drive than with the aims of (castrated) Eros.

Thus, we often see residents in the nursing home who split their object world with increasingly little stability between people and situations which signify death and nothingness, on the one hand, and others who "protect" them and keep them from falling in the cracks and holes forming in the Imaginary vase.[14] In this sense, we see in the fear of the final collapse into nothingness the last stand of Eros; similarly, all the primitive defenses like splitting, projection, envy and so on can be seen to be last stands of the defenses against the seduction of "nothingness"; or, to say this slightly differently, these defenses reflect a final defense of the barrier that Eros has erected between life and death.

And yet that is not all, or at least it need not be all. For the topic of nothingness brings up, in its train, the other topic of legacies. For if everything I have said in this chapter points in one direction it is toward the idea that the Real, the Imaginary, and the Symbolic of Lacan are all forms of desire that are also defenses against the subject's merging into nothingness precipitously, that is, as Freud said in *Beyond the Pleasure Principle* (1920), before the organism was naturally ready to die. The implication of this is that these forms of desire are, among other things, mental constructions designed to evade an encounter with nothingness, or, more specifically, they are constructions designed to help evade the desire of the subject for being nothing prematurely.

Part of *Hamlet*'s success as a play centers precisely on a Symbolic encounter with nothingness[15] of this sort; for, in the play, Hamlet is forced by the shocking return of his dead father, and by the prior violent actions of his uncle Claudius, and the equally violent desires of his mother, to come face to face with the nothingness of life; and, in fact, to do so while he was still unprepared, before his time, hence, in a way that traumatizes him.

Hamlet's untimely encounter with the ghost of his father acts as a trauma in the way trauma is described by Freud in *Beyond the Pleasure Principle* (1920). It paralyzes him and causes a compulsion to repeat the same thing over and over in a fashion that the playwright transforms into an inability to act. This may also remind some readers of Freud's discussion of Dostoevsky's childhood. You may recall that when he referred to the novelist, Freud stressed how the future writer was plagued by a premature death drive and by the fear he would be murdered by a vengeful father. The result of this premature exposure to death drives (along with a premature exposure to sexuality) was the guilty commandments emanating from a father imago in his unconscious. The reader may also recall that the Rat man also was haunted by hallucinations that he would murder his already dead father and his fiancée by inflicting the "rat torture" on them if he fulfilled a certain compulsive commandment to pay a certain Czech officer for his pince-nez. In other words, the obsessive reserve officer was also a victim of premature and excessive death drives that took the form of an encounter with a ghost. Finally, this train of thought may call to mind countless other deadly apparitions that appear in Freud's oeuvre.

Like these other encounters, Hamlet's father's ghost is a nothing that can still demand things from his hapless son. At the very least, it reminds Hamlet that he is fated to be a nothing like his father. In this sense, Hamlet's father is the return of the primal father; or to be even more exact, Hamlet's father's ghost marks the return of signifier for the return of the primal desire (really, manifested more in the figure of Claudius than Hamlet) that must be repressed by the Symbolic and substituted by the order of the Law.

Indeed, it is to avoid the need to act in a manner that this nothing-father-king demands that Hamlet feigns madness in the first place. That is, by feigning madness, Hamlet dithers and delays acting. But, in addition, by feigning to be mad, Hamlet maintains what little shred of civilization remains in Elsinore against the death drive in himself. Thus, according to this reading, it is when Hamlet is seemingly least effective and most seeming strange that he is truly upholding the Symbolic and Imaginary world that has crumbled all around him. Another way to say this is that by feigning madness Hamlet goes on living, and, in this manner, the Danish prince feigns that he has fallen into nothingness and gone mad in order to keep from completely being submerged by the nothingness reigning at Elsinore. Thus, Hamlet manages to hold the demand of his father-nothing at bay for a little while longer as his Eros demands and, in doing so, he rebels against the dead father by enacting a different sort of nothingness (a "staged nothingness" that mirrors the staging of the play) which nevertheless puts on stage for those with eyes to see the truth that the hidden structure of desire in the Danish court is mired in nothingness and blood-drenched death. Finally, in line with this interpretation, we can add the fact that Hamlet only gives in to the death drive in moments of true madness, first when he kills Polonius and than in the tragic sword fight at the play's end when he succumbs to an "inner madness."

To extend this further and to link it to our main subject, I would add that in the case of the residents and staff in the nursing home whom I have been discussing in this chapter, too, the demand that nothingness makes on them, and which they seek to avoid, is not a demand to revenge a dead father. Instead, it is a demand to embrace nothingness, to give in to their own prohibited desire to become nothing again, to break the final ties binding them to the living world.

And, it is at this point that the relation between nothingness and legacy begins to emerge more clearly. For, to feel one's self as being related to the Other is to feel oneself a part of something; whereas, to feel oneself as being cut off from the Other is to feel oneself to be nothing. Stating things in this manner may help us understand the extent to which all the defenses we have discussed, including the various structures of desire binding the subject to the Other, are all defenses against falling prematurely into nothingness by creating something. This applies to not only the formation of the neurotic subject but to every subject to the extent that the subject is a living subject, and we can include in this the Real, Imaginary, and Symbolic registers of the Lacanian subject of desire. In whatever form one wishes to conceive the formation of the subject, the coming into existence of a subject and its separation and knotting with the Other creates forms of desire that replace nothing with something.

And, hence, the problem that the collapse of the Symbolic and the Imaginary order reveals is that the ties that bind the subject to something are insufficient to represent reality in any but forms distorted by desire. And that is why simply reinforcing the resident's shaky Symbolic and Imaginary registers must also be insufficient to the task, too. Instead, a new kind of relation between the subject and the Other needs to be affirmed to resist a premature collapse into nothingness such as we saw in Hamlet's feigned madness and in the depression of many residents. This new form of desire needs to assert a connection between the subject and Other based on the idea of legacy which starts by acknowledging that each of us is burdened by a debt that we assume when we are born as quasi-sentient creatures and, as Freud knew when he associated that everyone owes life a death, everyone is weighed down by nothingness and the mortal structure of life—a mortal structure to life, however, that does not have to throw the subject into nothingness prematurely because he or she is also bound to eternity, or at least the subject remains bound to life, so long as the universe continues to reproduce and support organic life.

I will make some brief, concluding comments in the next, final chapter.

NOTES

1. Of course, no one experiences dying in the same way as the person next to them. Each person has his own preconscious and unconscious associations to death and aging. Thus, it always is X's or Y's (Imaginary) associations to the struggle against the satisfaction in things coming undone that counts. But, having said this, there obviously also are many points of commonality between the way individuals signify their drives. In this chapter I want to examine two specific defenses against the representations of death that frequently appear in nursing homes.

2. The picture is, in fact, more complicated at the drive level. Repetition compulsions of a painful and destructive sort are functioning here, too, such that splitting and negating also allow the compulsion to continue without entering directly into the conscious parts of the mind. As long ago as the 1930s, Ferenczi was defining this phenomena in the *Clinical Diary* as the psychic mark of trauma. The split-off part becomes a zone of the ego dominated by destructive death drives.

3. This depression, which may have a characterological base, reflects both the failure of the projective mechanism (the anger gets turned against the self) and the projection of anger against the "internal other or stranger." In this later form, the staff's depression also draws on associations to narcissistic wounds and fixations. On this later concept see Julia Kristeva, *Strangers to Ourselves*, trans. Leon S. Roudiez (New York: Columbia University Press, 1991); and, of course, respectively, Freud and Lacan on the structural role of castration in the unconscious.

4. This "distortion of reality" may be equated to the way an object (mass) warps or bends time and space, except in this case, it is reality, not time and space, that is bent and, in another sense, what is causing reality to bend is not the weight of a mass but the "weight" of having to live in a world already warped by castration anxiety and by the knowledge that we must die.

5. Between the 1920s and 1960s, Georges Bataille, Roger Caillois, Michel Leiris, and others influenced by Marcel Mauss' ethnography, Freudian psychoanalysis, Surrealism, and other avant-garde interests composed studies on public sacrifice and its literary-cultural and psychological-religious counterparts. Bataille uses the concept of the sacred to convey the altered state of consciousness produced in solitary individuals and crowds participating in spectacles of sacrifice. Rituals of sacrifice-death (human sacrifice, bull-fights, war, sexual frenzy, potlatches, writing) have the power to shatter the structures of time, order, and the Law and induce a Dionysian state of frenzy and fusion among onlookers, Bataille wrote, unleashing what Freud might have called an id frenzy. Bataille's aim was to undermine the groundwork of the moral self by replacing it with an unstable dialectic and materialist structures based on oscillating pairs such as the shit and purity, the sacred-profane, the "obscene part" and the Symbolic face of culture, and between heterogeny and homogeny. I might add that Bataille showed a keen interest in using the unconscious, surrealism, and the decentered subject as engines of war to destabilize the structures of the modern world and subject. His targets included most of the totalizing systems of his day, including capitalism, fascism, Marxism, Catholicism, aestheticism, and the other aspects of

what we might call the Symbolic structures of modern civilization and subjectivity. On these and related topics see Georges Bataille, *The Story of the Eye* (San Francisco: City Lights Publishers, 2001); Georges Bataille, *Visions of Excess: Selected Writings 1927–1939* (Minneapolis: University of Minnesota Press, 1985).

6. Michael Parson differentiates the defensive version of negation from a creative one, writing: "In his paper on negation Freud (1925) says clearly that negation is on the one hand defensive but also, on the other hand, important in freeing thinking from repression." Michael Parson, "Psychic Reality, Negation, and the Analytic Setting," in *The Dead Mother, The Work of Andre Green*, ed. Gregorio Kohon (London: Routledge, 1999).

7. It is less a case of simple laziness, therefore, than one of the staff needing to project sadistic impulses that the resident's helplessness arouses in them and so maintain distance from their own suffering.

8. Sandor Ferenczi, *The Clinical Diary of Sandor Ferenczi*, Judith Dupont, ed., (Cambridge, Mass.: Harvard University Press, 1995), 179.

9. This is Freud's definition of the death drive in *Beyond the Pleasure Principle*—the drive to die in order to return to an earlier state of inorganic rest.

10. Allen Ginsberg, "Father Death Blues," in *Collected Poems: 1947–1980* (New York: Harper's Perennial, 1988), 656.

11. The Real should not be misinterpreted as reality in the sense of the Kantian "ding-in-sich" or even the Freudian "reality principle." Instead the Real is the un- or the pre-representable register of the drives and of *jouissance*.

12. What this approach invites us to do is to not silence desire or to see it as nothing (at least to see it as nothing too precipitously), but, instead, to go into the structure of desire.

13. Lacan, Seminars, 324, quoted in Alenka Zupančič, "Ethics and Tragedy in Lacan," in *The Cambridge Companion to Lacan*, 256.

14. This sheds a new light on mythic narratives like the biblical story of Jonah that I will take up at a later time.

15. It, of course, also centers on an Imaginary encounter with "nothingness," especially in regards to Hamlet's relation to his mother, the Queen, and to other characters like Desdemona and her brother Laertes. Something similar can be said about Hamlet's relation to the Real, especially in his traumatic relation to his mother's *jouissance*. See Lacan's seminar on Hamlet.

10

Coda and Exit

Creon: "Stop being master now—the mastery you had in life has meant so little."

—Sophocles, *Oedipus Rex*

We have come to the end of this study of the death drive and the collapse into "nothingness" of residents in nursing homes. Before I finish, however, I want to ask one more question: it is whether or not we can draw a comparison between this fall into "nothingness" and the concepts of the "supplement," of "excess," of "the impossible," of "the accursed share," or of any number of other similar contemporary concepts. What I want to investigate, in short, is whether the collapse into "nothingness" and the struggle to maintain a structure of desire with "something" occurring in the nursing home does not have certain ethical and even, dare I say it, metapsychological weight.

Everyone knows that we do not go quietly into the night so long as there is any quantity of Eros left in us to resist death. People generally defy "flying into the falcon's beak" right up to the last moment of life. The problem is that the lives of the residents in the nursing home are often hell because the residents' libido is collapsing and their ties to the world around them are coming undone. I have examined this process of collapse of the Symbolic and Imaginary orders and, truthfully, the residents feel they are no longer master of their own bodies and lives but find this lack of mastery a final catastrophe.

This is the object-loss version of Freud's description in *Beyond the Pleasure Principle* (1920) of the life and death struggle of Eros to postpone the return to a state of non-being, where dying and death are the other side of the will to live and to put off the moment of truth. That much is indisputable. Freud does, however, more than say that a wish to die is the other side of the more "noisy" and conscious will to live. He shows, rather, that the will to live—the subject's will to build dams against the return to "nothingness"—is based on a defense against wanting to die. Lacan will modify this seminal idea by adding that the desire to live is also a structure of desire (really, the knotting together of three different structures of desire) binding the subject to the Other, and keeping the subject from its desire to return to a state of "nothingness." All the psychotic and neurotic-producing demands on the Other, and all the acceptance or rebellion against the necessity of living in a world where the Other enforces demands on us, can be seen as structures "to be" and to keep the subject from the desire to "not be."

In this sense, Lacan, via Freud, has modified Descartes' famous statement cogito ergo sum that grounds existence in thinking by the alternative construction: "I desire, so that I do not desire death." To switch to Kleinian terms like primitive projective mechanism, the child and adult projects his or her death drive to remove it from inside where it might draw the self to a premature death. The self will therefore project the drive toward self-destruction into internal object (but it also projects them into external objects, too), where the subject can relate to it as a foreign, dangerous, and, sometimes, seductive affect coming from a bad object via a paranoid attack. But on an ideological level, too, we might add we project our illusions of a bad world onto the bad object. We then can project ourselves or those whom we loved and hated into that world.

This is of a piece with the wish of the resident in the nursing home to disavow the possibility of their own death or to accept the loss of those they love (that is the work of mourning which can take many years to finish and often is never really begun by people who prefer to bury the pain of object loss and so consign their departed loved ones and hated enemies to a kind of psychological limbo). And yet, the slow or rapid collapse back to "nothingness" that we see in the nursing home is only an intensification and a culmination of processes occurring in everyone all the time, by which I mean that life is marred from its inception by tensions between maintaining life and bringing it to an end.

Thus, throughout their lives, people try to build up structures of desire, or ways of relating to the Other, to master or disavow the fundamentally traumatic and tragic structure to human existence; and this is the cause not only of the powerful urge in people to deny that they even have such a drive (to reach a state of non-being) which I have only been able to describe in a few cases in this book but also it is the cause of the tendency of people to distort reality in ways that gratify them. In old age, when the subject is forced to deal with one loss after the next, one affront to their narcissism after another, and a growing inability to protect themselves from the stimulation coming from the *jouissance* of the Other, their defenses are increasingly useless to them.

The question I want to raise before concluding this book is in what ways, and to what extent, is this defensive action against an inner drive to return to "nothingness" comparable to the way the subject and culture have been described by Bataille, Foucault, and others as something Derrida called the "supplement"? Derrida spoke of this supplement in quasi-psychological terms as being comparable to a symptom. A symptom is a disorder of some kind that appears in place of (as the representative of) something else that cannot appear. To say, therefore, that the supplement is comparable to a symptom is to infer that it is like a disorder of some kind that appears in the place of something else. But what can that something be? And why does the thing that appears in its place assume the form of a supplement?

Perhaps we could find some answers to this if we knew more about what Derrida meant by the term "supplement." The supplement, Derrida writes, appears "in order to designate something that can be neither assimilated nor rejected, neither internalized nor—since it transcends the boundary between internal/external—foreclosed."[1] This definition, I think, is most helpful in that it points us in a certain direction: the supplement is the "something" that appears in place of a "nothing," which is the best definition I can think of for "something that can be neither assimilated nor rejected"; but is it not a strange kind of "nothing" that is also something precisely because it cannot be assimilated or rejected? That is, it is a strange kind of "nothing" that has no place in any system, and for that very reason can guarantee the system by setting its outer limits, what is capable of being in the set of all sets comprising the system.

Unable to be assimilated or rejected, the "accursed share," as Bataille called it, has to fall under the bar of repression but, as Derrida writes, cannot be "foreclosed." What, we may ask, is this "accursed thing" that cannot be assimilated or rejected and, therefore, constantly returns from being expelled, repressed or simply "done away with" in the name of what is possible and impossible for the system? What is this thing that is "beyond good and evil"? What is this desire to become "nothing"? For, what else can this thing that has no place be, in the context of life, but death? And, what else can this thing be, in the context of a desiring subject existing in the midst of the structures of desire, except the desire for "nothingness" and non-being?

At any rate, we have seen throughout this book that, psychologically speaking, the thing that desire tries to unsuccessfully foreclose is the subject's desire for "nothingness"; and, apropos this, the Russian-born lecturer on Hegel in the thirties Alexandre Kojévé, who had such influence on Bataille's and Lacan's notion of negation of desire, made the self's refusal of "nothingness" the source of the slave's identity as slave. What this slave refuses is death, and so he loses the possibility of being a master. Instead, he acquiesces to the master who is master precisely because he is willing to risk everything up to and including death.

The point I want to bring out about this narrative is how Kojévé believed that life had to be lived in the full acknowledgement of the negative rather than be lived in the shadow of the refusal of death. Also, in the same collection of essays as the piece by Derrida on the supplement, Zizek writes, in a language that is more akin to that of Bataille, that the supplement is comparable to a "scandal and obscenity" undermining the subject's ongoing identifications with the Symbolic.[2]

Derrida also associates the symptom-supplement with the idea of "a foreign body to the ego."[3] And, one may be reminded here of the film *Invasion of the Body Snatchers* or perhaps the movie *Aliens*, but I hope that the concept of the supplement which is analogous to a foreign body also now reminds the reader of the residents he or she has read about in this book and especially of their feelings alienated from their bodies and of their struggles to hold on to a life in which the Symbolic and Imaginary bonds to the Other are coming undone.

Reading between the lines, we can say that the supplement that is being analyzed by Zizek and Derrida is a concept which is not really comparable to the death drive so much as it is something that is comparable to the symptom that appears in place of the death drive and which "ruins" our best laid plans and undermines the stability of the structures of desire that we build up over the course of a lifetime. There is, however, also a supplemental definition of the supplement that raises the question of the relation between the "wish to return to nothingness" and the ethical demand. You may recall that I briefly outlined an ethical stance that may arise from the collapse of the Imaginary and Symbolic orders into "nothingness" in a previous chapter. There, I said that the Imaginary and the Symbolic are built up as structures of desire that allow the subject to not acknowledge its desire for "nothingness" by replacing this desire with a desire for "something." But, once the Imaginary and Symbolic forms of desire are undermined, a new structure of desire can potentially emerge that springs from a place that acknowledges the death drive rather than from a place where the wish to return to "nothingness" is being disallowed ("foreclosed").

The question becomes how we begin to conceive of such a new law of desire that begins with acknowledging rather than with foreclosing the wish to become "nothing" to consciousness. Concepts like the supplement at least point us in the right direction. For Derrida, and Zizek even more forcefully, stresses that the subject normalizes (the violence of the Symbolic) while the symptom-supplement "decenters" it. And, being "something that can be neither assimilated nor rejected," the symptom-supplement is comparable to that "stone that gets stuck in the throat" discussed by Lacan in regards to the object a in *The Four Fundamental Concepts of Psychoanalysis*.[4] In this sense, the object a is a signifier of the "thing" that the supplement signifies that "can neither be assimilated nor rejected." That is, it is the representative of the subject's desire for non-being. It, therefore, is the thing that remains outside the system as non-normalizable, and, in terms of culture and life, the "accursed part," the despised stranger, the unwelcome return of the dead are all forms of the thing that cannot be assimilated.[5]

Should we then draw the comparison between these cultural concepts and what is happening to the minds of the residents in the nursing home whose ties to the Symbolic and Imaginary are collapsing? Are they, without necessarily wanting to, and certainly without being able to stop the process, being exposed to the final eruption of the "accursed share" too, as it undermines the structures of desire and overturns the final defenses against the return of the "impossible," the inassimilable wish to be "nothing"?

To answer this question, we need to return to *Beyond the Pleasure Principle* (1920) where Freud describes the drives as conservative. By calling the drives conservative he meant that their telos, even when the telos appears in the short term to be progressive and forward looking, is merely looking forward in order to find its way back, to reiterate, the past and to return to the original conflict between the drives and the environment at the dawn of life. As I said, when Freud made this assertion he was speaking about all the drives, both Eros and Thanatos, but he knew his assertion had special relevance to his discussion of the death drive since what he was arguing was that all the drives eventually are striving, in their own way, to return the organism to the state before life disturbed "nonbeing."

Freud knew, however, that the road back to the inorganic was blocked not only by the life drives but by the prior history of the clash between the life and death drives which left in its wake, pushed below the bar of repression and under "foreclosure," the remains of a catastrophe and a traumatic compulsion to repeat. The traumatic roots of psychic development not only pushed the ego to find different ways to live (to master the trauma) it also pulled the ego back toward repeating the trauma; and, beyond the trauma (although Freud was vaguer here) lies the uninhibited drive to be no more again. What this suggests is that (again, Freud was less clear on this than some others like Lacan have been) the catastrophe at the root of the ego also is the final defense against succumbing to the desire to become "nothing" again. For, the repetition compulsion of trauma that also figures so centrally in *Beyond the Pleasure Principle* (1920) besides the announcement of the death drive is merely, by being a repetition compulsion, a dam or barrier to the return to "nothingness."

Seeing this important connection between trauma, the compulsion to repeat, and the denial of the wish to return to the world of non-being not only helps clarify some of the comparisons between Freud's concept of the dual drive, Lacan's idea of the object a, and the notion of the symptom-supplement found in the articles by Zizek and Derrida, it also suggests a way to compare these rather esoteric ideas taken from the field of cultural studies and the collapse of the resident's mind into a longing for "nothingness." But we must be wary of making too much of such comparisons. For, it is extremely inappropriate and misguided to equate the suffering that the residents experience as the world that they knew begins to come undone to the epistemological debates of Derrida and the anti-aesthetic creative-destructive force that Bataille wrote about.

Building on modal and Aristotelian logic in his later investigation of feminine sexuality and *jouissance*, Lacan makes clear that he conceives of the mode of the "impossible," the "supplement," and "foreclosure" in very precise ways that do not conform to the connection between the death drive (the seduction of "nothingness") that I have made, and it may, therefore, be helpful to look more closely at some of the things Lacan said on this subject. To begin with, in an earlier discussion on Aristophanes' myth in the *Symposium*, Lacan develops a strange Imaginary character that he calls the *lamella*. The *lamella*, Lacan says, corresponds to the bit of sexuality that is cut off and lost when Zeus (you will recall the story I told in the opening chapter of this book) divides human beings in two. The *lamella*, then, signifies a mythic (possible, Imaginary) representation of that part of sexuality and being that humanity can no longer access after they enter the Symbolic world, that is when they become creatures whose being is defined by language. The *lamella* is, at once, the lost trace of the natural world that human beings are forever cut off from at the same time as it is the primal object of desire that can never be represented (without leaving the world of the natural and entering into the world of the Symbolic); hence, it is at once the object a, the representation of the thing that cannot be represented and remain itself (the "impossible"), the surplus, excess, and supplement to discourse that Derrida mentions, and the thing to which access is forever "foreclosed"—incestuous and murderous *jouissance*.

We have to be clear: this is not the same use of the word "foreclosure" that appears in Lacan's study of Freud's three forms of negation where Lacan says negation has three forms corresponding to the clinical categories of the neurosis, perversion, and psychosis. In essence, the neurotic (the hysteric especially) denies what is known by means of repressing the knowledge into the unconscious. The pervert disavows the knowledge (he both knows it and does not know it), the principal example of this being the way a sexual pervert knows and does not know that the woman does not have a penis. Finally, "foreclosure" is a far more radical form of negation associated by Lacan to psychosis in which the Symbolic world is being denied for an individual one. And yet, in some respects, without being psychotic, the residents who are losing their attachments to the Symbolic and Imaginary order are moving back toward a kind of "foreclosure" where the last ties to a representational reality are being dominated by death drives and by representations of death and dying.

But to return to our problem, Lacan clearly imagines the *lamella* to be a part of libido and sexuality and not a part of the death drive. Similarly, when Lacan comes to modify the notion that there is only phallic (masculine) libido in his essay on "feminine sexuality" he clearly wants to associate the possibility of an evanescent, fleeting mode of female sexuality and *jouissance* with there also being a possible (because pertaining to the mode of the contingent rather than the universal) way to gain access to a "surplus excess," or a "supplement," that is forbidden to and foreclosed by the Symbolic.

But how can one gain access to this state of being "beyond the discursive," while one admits, as Lacan does, that one cannot "think" outside of the discursive, and, hence, one cannot think "beyond" without making it a part of the Symbolic world it is seeking to transcend? Perhaps Lacan points us in the right direction when he writes his famous square of "sexuation," which I can only refer to briefly and in passing. For in his discussion of sexuation, Lacan says the opposite number of the Symbolic is the "impossible," and he then finds in Freud's "Totem and Taboo" the mythic expression of this relation, for, Lacan says, in Freud's mythos, the Symbolic order can only come into being by "foreclosing" and excluding the unlimited *jouissance* of the primal father; that is to say, when the brothers killed the primal father, they did so in order to seize his unlimited *jouissance* for themselves, but in order to live with each other, all the brothers had to Symbolically renounce that desire; and so, they entered the Symbolic by collectively accepting being cut off (castrated) from a piece of being: the desire for the *jouissance* of the death drive.

The important thing for Lacan is that a part of *jouissance* and libido is lost when humans left the state of nature and developed language and this piece of existence is foreclosed to us. But Freud (perhaps more emphatically than Lacan) said that it is not just a piece of libido that the brothers abandoned when they entered the Symbolic order, it was also a drive to destroy that they had to forbid themselves and which they had to bury beneath an unending number of Symbolic substitutions until the day finally came when their remaining libido was no longer able to hold back the old drive, the desire for "nothingness."

And, is this not what happens in the minds of the residents who are losing their libido and their Symbolic and Imaginary attachments that defend them against their own drive to destroy and eventually to return to "nothingness" (by making them replace the original wish by more or less effective substitutions)?

I say this with the greatest hesitancy, however, since I am the last person to know what such a relation to being would be, except that, whatever it is, it involves the subject's relations to the urge to destroy (and ultimately for "nothingness") which Lacan associates with the drive as much as it involves the forms of sexuality and libido; or, to be more precise, I think a close reading of Lacan shows (and this is even more emphatically the case with Freud) that the forms libido assumes (the forms of the wish) are, at their most basic level, knotted up with the drive to escape from the drive to be "nothing" again.

This, of course, describes the inner world of the residents I have described in this book who, as a group, are in various states of unending mourning. But, Lacan shows us (Freud did too, of course, but Lacan often does it more emphatically) that we are *all* inescapably tied to mourning loss endlessly, because we are creatures of language, first of all, and, therefore, creatures of desire and Symbolic exchange who are forever cut off from nature. So, tying this notion of perpetual mourning to the discussion above on the emergence of the Symbolic order out the "foreclosure" of a piece of libido tied to the urgings of the death drive, I cannot help but return to Freud's comments near the end of his essay "On Transience" (1915) where he exclaims to no one and to everyone: "Would it not be better to give death the place in reality and in our thoughts that is its due, and bring out the unconscious attitudes to death, which we have hitherto so carefully suppressed, a little more?"[6] Or, when that is not feasible (which it often is not), as is often the case of older residents, then we can perhaps guide them to an easier passage, where their loss does not leave them bereft of Eros and comfort from the other. Ultimately, the best we can do (but it already is a lot) in many cases is to provide love (we give our Eros to them). For, if psychoanalytic research teaches us one thing, it is this: that we are inescapably bound to the Symbolic order (we cannot think without words, and hence our only access to being is through words), but the Symbolic ties us to the rock of castration since we have had to lose a piece of being (nature) that is forever foreclosed to us. As early as his 1915 essays on war, death, and mourning, Freud wonders why people hold on to their grief and do not return to the world able to love again. That is to say, he wonders what has happened to their libido? This is not as naïve a question as it seems if we just consider, to take only one problem, how in mourning both object-love and narcissistic-love are deeply impaired and the ego can only express its abiding attachment to the (lost) object by berating itself and harming itself by cutting itself off from any new attachments (which as we saw in previous chapters is the vital ingredient to a person either not getting sick or recovering from illness). And, faced with this problem (what has happened to the libido of the person who cannot find love again), Freud concludes that such people are burdened because "something is blocking the flow of their libido so, their revolt against grief" devalues "the pleasure of beautiful things for them."[7]

Hence, we are forever mourning. But more than this, psychoanalytic research shows us that our way of relating to the Symbolic world, the various manners we desire the other as subjects are substitutions that began in the act of loss, and before that, in the act of giving ourselves over to our death drives. The entire Symbolic and Imaginary orders, therefore, are rooted in this wish to find substitute forms of desire to express our guilt (Freud) or our loss (Lacan) and to foreclose our direct experience of the desire for "nothingness" again.

The Symbolic therefore has a history, and it has formed out of a need to deny the death drive and the guilt and loss that it wrought. If there is a way forward to a new form of desire that is not stuck in the Law (formed to stop the return of the death drive), that is not locked into the morality of the superego, then it will require the subject to take up a new relation to death and to its own (forbidden) death drive. If we can do that, we will bring a little more truth into our relation to ourselves and to others which can, in the end, only have positive effects on the way we treat one another.

The thought of death is hard, but it turns out that acknowledging an inward drive to "nothingness" is even harder to accept. But, in the end, if we do not acknowledge our true desires how can we make peace with ourselves and with the other and so, if not bring the trauma at the root of existence to an end, at least allow us to relate to the other in a more humane way? At the center of this more human attitude to the other will be an acceptance that we both want and do not want to be "nothing" again and that we want and do not want to push others into a state of "nothingness" so that we can go on living for a little while longer; and, this will place us in a new sort of relation to the Other and force us to reconsider our attachments to all the others who have made us who we are, and who have defined with us the structure of our desires.

In sum, if, as Dylan Thomas wrote, we do not go softly into the night, we can at least bear our desires for "nothingness" a little better.

NOTES

1. Derrida, "Geopsychoanalysis: '. . . and the rest of the world,'" in *The Psychoanalysis of Race*, ed. Christophe Lane (New York: Columbia University Press,

1998), 68. We might supplement this commentary by saying that it cannot be foreclosed—except in death.

2. Slavoj Zizek, "Love thy Neighbor? No thanks!" in *The Psychoanalysis of Race*, 154–75.

3. The reader understands that Derrida is not a Lacanian and so he does not make the distinction between the ego, the self, and the subject that is so vital to Lacan. In this instance, "ego" simply means the internal sense of "I" that a person carries around in their head.

4. Psychoanalytically, this set might include anxiety of castration, object loss, incestuous fantasy, bisexuality, and murderous wishes expressive of the death drive.

5. Besides concepts like the narcissism of small differences, Freud already drew attention to the association of stranger and the despised in "Totem and Taboo" (1912–1913). This notion has been developed in the work of many contemporary French thinkers including Levinas. It also has become central to the project of Kristeva; and, along with Kristeva, Derrida associates this foreign body with the "ostracized stranger." Kristeva, *Strangers to Ourselves*, Leon S. Roudiez, trans. (New York: Columbia University Press, 1994). This entire way of speaking and thinking, of course, has roots in Europe's Romantic and Idealist traditions, and, in particular, its vision of Being as becoming, or as Bataille says—excess, as something that is constantly creating the new and leaving the old form behind like a dead husk. In line with this thinking, however, death is not just a passive—nevermore—but is an active participant with creativity, clearing away the old for the new.

6. Freud writes: "Death can no longer be denied."

7. Freud, "On Transience," 198.

Bibliography

Abraham, K. (1978). *Le Complexe de Castration: Un Fantasme Originaire*. Paris, Tchou.

Akhtar, S. (2001). *Three Faces of Mourning: Melancholia, Manic Defense, and Moving On*. Northvale, N.J., Jason Aronson.

Alcorn, M. W. (1994). *Narcissism and the Literary Libido: Rhetoric, Text, and Subjectivity*. New York, New York University Press.

Alford, C. F. (1991). *The Self in Social Theory: A Psychoanalytic Account of Its Construction in Plato, Hobbes, Locke, Rawls, and Rousseau*. New Haven, Conn., Yale University Press.

Althusser, L. (1993). *Ecrits sur la Psychanalyse: Freud et Lacan*. France, Stock/IMEC.

Althusser, L., and F. Matheron (2003). *The Humanist Controversy and Other Writings, 1966–1967*. London; New York, Verso.

Assoun, P. L. (2000). *Freud and Nietzsche*. London; New Brunswick, N.J. Somerset, N.J., Athlone Press; Distributed in the U.S. by Transaction Publishers.

Badiou, A. (2008). *Conditions*. London; New York, Continuum.

Bass, A. (2000). *Difference and Disavowal: The Trauma of Eros*. Stanford, Calif., Stanford University Press.

Bataille, G. (1972). *Le Procès de Gilles De Rais*. Paris, J. J. Pauvert.

Bataille, G. (1977). *Death and Sensuality: A Study of Eroticism and the Taboo*. New York, Arno Press.

Bataille, G. (1977). *Sade*. Paris, Obliques.

Bataille, G. (1978). *Blue of Noon*. New York, Urizen Books.

Bataille, G. (1988). *The Accursed Share: An Essay on General Economy*. New York, Zone Books.

Bataille, G., and D. Hollier (1988). *The College of Sociology (1937–39)*. Minneapolis, University of Minnesota Press.

Bataille, G., and B. Noël (1967). *La Pratique de la Joie Devant la Mort*. Paris, Mercure de France.

Baudrillard, J. (1993). *Symbolic Exchange and Death*. London; Thousand Oaks, Sage Publications.

Benjamin, J. (1998). *Shadow of the Other: Intersubjectivity and Gender in Psychoanalysis*. New York, Routledge.

Bergmann, M. S. (2000). *The Hartmann Era*. New York, The Other Press.

Blanchot, M., E. Rottenberg, et al. (2000). *The Instant of My Death*. Stanford, Calif., Stanford University Press.

Bloch, D. (1994). *So the Witch Won't Eat Me: Fantasy and the Child's Fear of Infanticide*. Northvale, N.J., Jason Aronson.

Breger, L. (2000). *Freud: Darkness in the Midst of Vision*. New York, Wiley.

Britton, R. (2003). *Sex, Death, and the Super-Ego: Experiences in Psychoanalysis*. London; New York, Karnac.

Brooks, P., and A. Woloch (2000). *Whose Freud?: The Place of Psychoanalysis in Contemporary Culture*. New Haven, Conn., Yale University Press.

Brown, N. O. (1985). *Life Against Death: The Psychoanalytical Meaning of History*. Middletown, Conn.; Scranton, Pa., Wesleyan University Press; Distributed by Harper & Row.

Chasseguet-Smirgel, J. (1984). *Creativity and Perversion*. New York, W.W. Norton.

Chasseguet-Smirgel, J. (1985). *The Ego Ideal: A Psychoanalytic Essay on the Malady of the Ideal*. London, Free Association Books.

Copjec, J. (1994). *Supposing the Subject*. London; New York, Verso.

De Masi, F. (2004). *Making Death Thinkable: A Psychoanalytic Contribution to the Problem of the Transience of Life*. London, Free Association Books.

Derrida, J. (1995). *The Gift of Death*. Chicago, University of Chicago Press.

Derrida, J. (2007). *Psyche: Inventions of the Other*. Stanford, Calif., Stanford University Press.

Dever, C. (1998). *Death and the Mother from Dickens to Freud: Victorian Fiction and the Anxiety of Origins*. Cambridge; New York, Cambridge University Press.

Dietrich, D. R., and P. C. Shabad (1989). *The Problem of Loss and Mourning: Psychoanalytic Perspectives*. Madison, Conn., International Universities Press.

Dollimore, J. (1998). *Death, Desire, and Loss in Western Culture*. New York, Routledge.

Drassinower, A. (2003). *Freud's Theory of Culture: Eros, Loss, and Politics*. Lanham, Md., Rowman & Littlefield Publishers.

Eigen, M. (1996). *Psychic Deadness*. Northvale, N.J., Jason Aronson.

Einstein, A., S. Freud, et al. (1933). *Why War?* [Paris], International Institute of Intellectual Co-Operation, League of Nations.

Elliott, A. (1996). *Subject to Ourselves: Social Theory, Psychoanalysis, and Postmodernity*. Cambridge, Mass., Polity Press.

Fairfield, S., L. Layton, et al. (2002). *Bringing the Plague: Toward Postmodern Psychoanalysis*. New York, The Other Press.

Ferenczi, S. (1980). *Final Contributions to the Problems and Methods of Psycho-Analysis*. New York, Brunner/Mazel.

Ferenczi, S., and J. Dupont (1988). *The Clinical Diary of Sándor Ferenczi*. Cambridge, Mass., Harvard University Press.

Ferenczi, S., G. Groddeck, et al. (1982). *Correspondance (1921–1933)*. Paris, Payot.

Forter, G., and P. A. Miller (2008). *Desire of the Analysts: Psychoanalysis and Cultural Criticism*. Albany, State University of New York Press.

Frankiel, R. V. (1994). *Essential Papers on Object Loss*. New York, New York University Press.

Freud, S. (2002). *"The Wolfman" and Other Cases*. London, Penguin.

Freud, S. (2003). *The Psychopathology of Everyday Life*. New York, Penguin Books.

Freud, S., L. Andreas-Salomé, et al. (1970). *Correspondance [De Lou Andreas Salomé]*. Paris, Gallimard.

Freud, S., and J. Crick (2002). *The Joke and Its Relation to the Unconscious*. London; New York, Penguin.

Freud, S., S. Ferenczi, et al. (1993). *The Correspondence of Sigmund Freud and Sándor Ferenczi*. Cambridge, Mass., Belknap Press of Harvard University Press.

Freud, S., G. Fichtner, et al. (2003). *The Sigmund Freud-Ludwig Binswanger Correspondence 1908–1938*. New York, The Other Press.

Freud, S., J. M. Masson, et al. (1985). *The Complete Letters of Sigmund Freud to Wilhelm Fliess, 1887–1904*. Cambridge, Mass., Belknap Press of Harvard University Press.

Freud, S., D. Mclintock, et al. (2003). *The Uncanny*. New York, Penguin Books.

Freud, S., J. Sandler, et al. (1991). *On Freud's "Analysis Terminable and Interminable."* New Haven, Conn., Yale University Press.

Freud, S., and D. H. Spain (1992). *Psychoanalytic Anthropology After Freud: Essays Marking the Fiftieth Anniversary of Freud's Death*. New York, Psyche Press.

Freud, S., J. Strachey, et al. (1953). *The Standard Edition of the Complete Psychological Works of Sigmund Freud*. London, Hogarth Press.

Freud, S., and S. Whiteside (2007). *The Psychology of Love*. New York, Penguin Books.

Freud, S., A. Zweig, et al. (1987). *The Letters of Sigmund Freud and Arnold Zweig*. New York, New York University Press.

Frosh, S. (1991). *Identity Crisis: Modernity, Psychoanalysis, and the Self*. New York, Routledge.

Fryer, D. R. (2009). *Thinking Queerly: Race, Sex, Gender, and the Ethics of Identity*. Boulder, Colo., Paradigm Publishers.

Gambaudo, S. (2007). *Kristeva, Psychoanalysis and Culture: Subjectivity in Crisis*. Aldershot, England; Burlington, Vt., Ashgate.

Gantt, E. E., and R. N. Williams (2002). *Psychology for the Other: Levinas, Ethics, and the Practice of Psychology*. Pittsburgh, Duquesne University Press.

Geyskens, T., and P. V. Haute (2007). *From Death Instinct to Attachment Theory: The Primacy of the Child in Freud, Klein and Hermann*. New York, The Other Press.

Gherovici, P. (2003). *The Puerto Rican Syndrome*. New York, The Other Press.

Gillespie, W. H., M. D. A. Sinason, Et al. (1995). *Life, Sex, and Death: Selected Writings of William H. Gillespie*. London; New York, Routledge.

Glick, R. A., and D. I. Meyers (1988). *Masochism: Current Psychoanalytic Perspectives*. Hillsdale, N.J., Analytic Press: Distributed by Lawrence Erlbaum.

Goodwin, S. M. W., and E. Bronfen (1993). *Death and Representation*. Baltimore, Johns Hopkins University Press.

Gray, W. (2008). *Death and Fantasy: Essays on Philip Pullman, C.S. Lewis, George Macdonald, and R.L. Stevenson*. Newcastle Upon Tyne, UK, Cambridge Scholars Pub.

Green, A. (1999). *The Work of the Negative*. London; New York, Free Association Books.

Green, A. (2007). *Pourquoi les Pulsions de Destruction ou de Mort?* Paris, Panama.

Grigg, R. (2008). *Lacan, Language, and Philosophy*. Albany, NY, State University of New York Press.

Grunberger, B., and J. Chasseguet-Smirgel (1986). *Freud or Reich?: Psychoanalysis and Illusion*. New Haven, Conn., Yale University Press.

Grunberger, B., and D. Macey (1989). *New Essays on Narcissism*. London, Free Association Books.

Guntrip, H. (1968). *Schizoid Phenomena, Object-Relations, and the Self*. New York, International Universities Press.

Gurewich, J. F., M. Tort, et al. (1996). *The Subject and the Self: Lacan and American Psychoanalysis*. Northvale, N.J., Jason Aronson.

Güven, F. (2005). *Madness and Death in Philosophy*. Albany, State University of New York Press.

Hägglund, T. B. (1978). *Dying: A Psychoanalytic Study with Special Reference to Individual Creativity and Defensive Organization*. New York, International Universities Press.

Harari, R. (2004). *Lacan's Four Fundamental Concepts of Psychoanalysis: An Introduction*. New York, The Other Press.

Haute, P. V. (2002). *Against Adaptation: Lacan's "Subversion of the Subject."* New York, The Other Press.

Holbrook, D. (1971). *Human Hope and the Death Instinct: An Exploration of Psychoanalytical Theories of Human Nature and their Implications for Culture and Education*. Oxford; New York, Pergamon Press.

Hughes, J. M. (2007). *Guilt and Its Vicissitudes: Psychoanalytic Reflections on Morality*. Hove, East Sussex; New York, Routledge.

Hurst, A. (2008). *Derrida Vis-à-Vis Lacan: Interweaving Deconstruction and Psychoanalysis*. New York, Fordham University Press.

Irigaray, L. (1993). *An Ethics of Sexual Difference*. Ithaca, N.Y., Cornell University Press.

Iversen, M. (2007). *Beyond Pleasure: Freud, Lacan, Barthes*. University Park, Pa., Pennsylvania State University Press.

Jung, C. G., and J. L. Yates (1999). *Jung on Death nd Immortality*. Princeton, N.J., Princeton University Press.

Kernberg, O. F. (1975). *Borderline Conditions and Pathological Narcissism*. New York, Jason Aronson.

Kernberg, O. F. (1992). *Aggression in Personality Disorders and Perversions*. New Haven, Conn., Yale University Press.

Khan, M. M. R. (1974). *The Privacy of the Self*. London, Hogarth Press [For] The Institute of Psycho-Analysis.

Klein, M. (1975). *Envy and Gratitude, and Other Works, 1946–1963*. London, Hogarth Press and The Institute Of Psycho-Analysis.

Klein, M. (1984). *Love, Guilt, and Reparation, and Other Works, 1921–1945*. New York, Free Press.

Klein, M., and J. Mitchell (1987). *The Selected Melanie Klein*. New York, Free Press.

Kohon, G. (1999). *The Dead Mother: The Work of André Green*. New York, Routledge.

Kohut, H. (2009). *The Restoration of the Self*. Chicago, The University of Chicago Press.

Kristeva, J. (1991). *Strangers to Ourselves*. New York, Columbia University Press.

Kristeva, J. (1995). *New Maladies of the Soul*. New York, Columbia University Press.

Lacan, J. (1978). *The Four Fundamental Concepts of Psycho-Analysis*. New York, Norton.

Lacan, J. (1992). *The Ethics of Psychoanalysis, 1959–1960*. New York, Norton.

Lacan, J. (2006). *The Other Side of Psychoanalysis*. New York, Norton.

Lacan, J., and B. Fink (2006). *Ecrits: The First Complete Edition in English*. New York, W.W. Norton & Co.

Lacan, J., and J. A. Miller (1988). *The Seminar of Jacques Lacan*. New York, Norton.

Laplanche, J. (1976). *Life and Death in Psychoanalysis*. Baltimore, Johns Hopkins University Press.

Laplanche, J., and J. Fletcher (1999). *Essays on Otherness*. London; New York, Routledge.

Lear, J. (2000). *Happiness, Death, and the Remainder of Life*. Cambridge, Mass., Harvard University Press.

Leclaire, S. (1998). *A Child Is Being Killed: On Primary Narcissism and the Death Drive*. Stanford, Calif., Stanford University Press.

Lefort, R., and R. Lefort (1994). *Birth of the Other*. Urbana, University of Illinois Press.

Lévinas, E. (1998). *Entre Nous: On Thinking-of-the-Other*. New York, Columbia University Press.

Limentani, A. (1998). *Between Freud and Klein: The Psychoanalytic Quest for Knowledge and Truth*. London, Karnac Books.

Marcus, P. (2008). *Being for the Other: Emmanuel Levinas, Ethical Living and Psychoanalysis*. Milwaukee, Wisc., Marquette University Press.

Marcuse, H. (1969). *Eros and Civilization: A Philosophical Inquiry into Freud*. London, Sphere.

Muensterberger, W. (1970). *Man and His Culture: Psychoanalytic Anthropology after "Totem and Taboo."* New York, Taplinger Pub. Co.

Nobus, D., and M. Quinn (2005). *Knowing Nothing, Staying Stupid: Elements for a Psychoanalytic Epistemology*. London; New York, Routledge.

Person, E. S., P. Fonagy, et al. (1995). *On Freud's "Creative Writers and Day-Dreaming."* New Haven, Conn., Yale University Press.

Person, E. S., S. Freud, et al. (1997). *On Freud's "A Child Is Being Beaten."* New Haven, Conn., Yale University Press.

Person, E. S., A. Hagelin, et al. (1993). *On Freud's "Observations on Transference-Love."* New Haven, Conn., Yale University Press.

Piven, J. S. (2004). *Death and Delusion: A Freudian Analysis of Mortal Terror*. Greenwich, U.K., IAP.

Plon, M., and H. Rey-Flaud (2004). *La Pulsion de Mort Entre Psychanalyse et Philosophie*. Ramonville Saint-Agne, France, Erès.

Quinodoz, D. (2009). *Growing Old: A Journey of Self-Discovery*. New York, Routledge.

Rabaté, J. M. (2003). *The Cambridge Companion to Lacan*. Cambridge, U.K.; New York, Cambridge University Press.

Ragland-Sullivan, E. (1995). *Essays on the Pleasures of Death: From Freud to Lacan*. New York, Routledge.

Rank, O. (1993). *The Trauma of Birth*. New York, Dover.

Ray, N. (2009). *Tragedy and Otherness: Sophocles, Shakespeare, Psychoanalysis*. Oxford; New York, Peter Lang.

Reik, T. (1957). *Myth and Guilt: The Crime and Punishment of Mankind*. New York, G. Braziller.

Ricciardi, A. (2003). *The Ends of Mourning: Psychoanalysis, Literature, Film*. Stanford, Calif., Stanford University Press.

Rosenthal, L. (1987). *Resolving Resistance in Group Psychotherapy*. Northvale, N.J., Jason Aronson.

Rudnytsky, P. L. (1993). *Transitional Objects and Potential Spaces: Literary Uses of D.W. Winnicott*. New York, Columbia University Press.

Rudnytsky, P. L., and E. H. Spitz (1994). *Freud and Forbidden Knowledge*. New York, New York University Press.

Safranski, R. (1998). *Martin Heidegger: Between Good and Evil*. Cambridge, Mass., Harvard University Press.

Safranski, R. (2002). *Nietzsche: A Philosophical Biography*. New York, W.W. Norton.

Sanchez-Pardo, E. (2003). *Cultures of the Death Drive: Melanie Klein and Modernist Melancholia*. Durham, N.C., Duke University Press.

Sartre, J. P. (1988). *Mallarmé, or, the Poet of Nothingness*. University Park, Pennsylvania State University Press.

Schmidt-Hellerau, C. (2001). *Life Drive & Death Drive, Libido & Lethe: A Formalized Consistent Model of Psychoanalytic Drive and Structure Theory*. New York, The Other Press.

Shengold, L. (1991). *"Father, Don't You See I'm Burning?": Reflections on Sex, Narcissism, Symbolism, and Murder: From Everything to Nothing*. New Haven, Conn., Yale University Press.

Siegel, A. M. (1996). *Heinz Kohut and the Psychology of the Self*. London; New York, Routledge.

Solms, M., and O. Turnbull (2002). *The Brain and the Inner World: An Introduction to the Neuroscience of Subjective Experience*. New York, The Other Press.

Spotnitz, H. (1999). *Modern Psychoanalysis of the Schizophrenic Patient: Theory of the Technique*. Northvale, N.J., Jason Aronson.

Spotnitz, H., and P. W. Meadow (1995). *Treatment of the Narcissistic Neuroses*. Northvale, N.J., Jason Aronson.

Stepansky, P. E. (1977). *A History of Aggression in Freud*. New York, International Universities Press.

Stolorow, R. D. (1993). *Faces in a Cloud: Intersubjectivity in Personality Theory*. Northvale, N.J., Jason Aronson.

Verhaeghe, P. (2009). *New Studies of Old Villains: A Radical Reconsideration of the Oedipus Complex*. New York, The Other Press.

Volkan, V. D. (1976). *Primitive Internalized Object Relations: A Clinical Study of Schizophrenic, Borderline, and Narcissistic Patients*. New York, International Universities Press.

Voruz, V., and B. Wolf (2007). *The Later Lacan: An Introduction*. Albany, State University of New York Press.

Weatherill, R. (1999). *The Death Drive: New Life for a Dead Subject?* London, Rebus Press.

Weininger, O. (1996). *Being and Not Being: Clinical Applications of the Death Instinct*. Madison, Conn., International Universities Press.

Wellings, N., and E. W. Mccormick (2005). *Nothing to Lose: Psychotherapy, Buddhism and Living Life*. London; New York, Continuum. Press: Institute of Psycho-Analysis.

Winnicott, D. W. (1986). *Holding and Interpretation: Fragment of an Analysis*. London, Hogarth.

Winnicott, D. W., C. Winnicott, et al. (1989). *Psycho-Analytic Explorations*. Cambridge, Mass., Harvard University Press.

Yerushalmi, Y. H., and S. Freud (1991). *Freud's Moses: Judaism Terminable and Interminable*. New Haven, Conn., Yale University Press.

Zizek, S. (1994). *The Metastases of Enjoyment: Six Essays on Woman and Causality*. London; New York, Verso.

Zizek, S. (2008). *Violence: Six Sideways Reflections*. New York, Picador.

Index

About the Author

Andrew Stein received a Ph.D. in Modern European History in 1993. Subsequent to that, he received a second Ph.D. in Clinical Psychology in 2004 and has finished training as a Modern Psychoanalyst. He currently resides in New York City, where he sees patients in private practice and at a number of nursing home facilities.

Breinigsville, PA USA
10 January 2010
230465BV00003B/6/P

9 780765 705778